C

Endocrine and
Reproductive
Systems

One Stop Doc

Titles in the series include:

Cardiovascular System – Jonathan Aron
Editorial Advisor – Jeremy Ward

Cell and Molecular Biology – Desikan Rangarajan and David Shaw
Editorial Advisor – Barbara Moreland

Gastrointestinal System – Miruna Canagaratnam
Editorial Advisor – Richard Naftalin

Musculoskeletal System – Wayne Lam, Bassel Zebian and Rishi Aggarwal
Editorial Advisor – Alistair Hunter

Nervous System – Elliott Smock
Editorial Advisor – Clive Coen

Metabolism and Nutrition – Miruna Canagaratnam and David Shaw
Editorial Advisor – Barbara Moreland and Richard Naftalin

Renal and Urinary System and Electrolyte Balance – Panos Stamoulos and Spyros Bakalis
Editorial Advisor – Richard Naftalin and Alistair Hunter

Respiratory System – Jo Dartnell and Michelle Ramsay
Editorial Advisor – John Rees

ONE STOP DOC

Endocrine and Reproductive Systems

Caroline Jewels BSc (Hons)
Fifth year medical student, Guy's, King's and
St Thomas' Medical School, London, UK

Alexandra Tillet BSc (Hons)
Fifth year medical student, Guy's, King's and
St Thomas' Medical School, London, UK

Editorial Advisor: Stuart Milligan MA DPHIL
Professor of Reproductive Biology, Department of Physiology,
Guy's, King's and St Thomas' School of Biomedical Sciences, King's College, London, UK

Series Editor: Elliott Smock BSc (Hons)
Fifth year medical student, Guy's, King's and
St Thomas' Medical School, London, UK

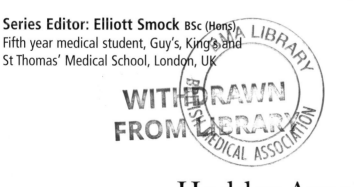

Hodder Arnold

A MEMBER OF THE HODDER HEADLINE GROUP

First published in Great Britain in 2005 by
Hodder Education, a member of the Hodder Headline Group,
338 Euston Road, London NW1 3BH

http://www.hoddereducation.co.uk

Distributed in the United States of America by
Oxford University Press Inc.,
198 Madison Avenue, New York, NY10016
Oxford is a registered trademark of Oxford University Press

Whilst the advice and information in this book are believed to be true and
accurate at the date of going to press, neither the authors nor the publisher
can accept any legal responsibility or liability for any errors or omissions
that may be made. In particular (but without limiting the generality of the
preceding disclaimer) every effort has been made to check drug dosages;
however it is still possible that errors have been missed. Furthermore,
dosage schedules are constantly being revised and new side-effects
recognized. For these reasons the reader is strongly urged to consult the
drug companies' printed instructions before administering any of the drugs
recommended in this book.

British Library Cataloguing in Publication Data
A catalogue record for this book is available from the British Library

Library of Congress Cataloging-in-Publication Data
A catalog record for this book is available from the Library of Congress

ISBN-10: 0 340 885068
ISBN-13: 978 0 340 88506 2

1 2 3 4 5 6 7 8 9 10

Commissioning Editor: Georgina Bentliff
Project Editor: Heather Smith
Production Controller: Jane Lawrence
Cover Design: Amina Dudhia
Illustrations: Cactus Design

Typeset in 10/12pt Adobe Garamond/Akzidenz GroteskBE by Servis Filmsetting Ltd, Manchester
Printed and bound in Spain

Hodder Headline's policy is to use papers that are natural, renewable and recyclable products
and made from wood grown in sustainable forests. The logging and manufacturing processes
are expected to conform to the environmental regulations of the country of origin.

What do you think about this book? Or any other Hodder Arnold title?
Please visit our website at **www.hoddereducation.co.uk**

CONTENTS

PREFACE

From the Series Editor, Elliott Smock

Are you ready to face your looming exams? If you have done loads of work, then congratulations; we hope this opportunity to practice SAQs, EMQs, MCQs and Problem-based Questions on every part of the core curriculum will help you consolidate what you've learnt and improve your exam technique. If you don't feel ready, don't panic – the One Stop Doc series has all the answers you need to catch up and pass.

There are only a limited number of questions an examiner can throw at a beleaguered student and this text can turn that to your advantage. By getting straight into the heart of the core questions that come up year after year and by giving you the model answers you need this book will arm you with the knowledge to succeed in your exams. Broken down into logical sections, you can learn all the important facts you need to pass without having to wade through tons of different textbooks when you simply don't have the time. All questions presented here are 'core'; those of the highest importance have been highlighted to allow even shaper focus if time for revision is running out. In addition, to allow you to organize your revision efficiently, questions have been grouped by topic, with answers supported by detailed integrated explanations.

On behalf of all the One Stop Doc authors I wish you the very best of luck in your exams and hope these books serve you well!

From the Authors, Caroline Jewels and Alexandra Tillett

Writing a book during our final year was quite an undertaking, but is has been hugely rewarding. Getting through medical school exams is no easy task. Hopefully, this book will provide you with a good understanding of the basic concepts of endocrinology and reproductive physiology that you can use tirelessly in the future, impressing tutors and clinicians alike. If not, then at least it may provide you with the ability to sit (and pass!) pre-clinical exams.

Chapters have been logically divided into key topics that you WILL be tested on. We have provided detailed explanations in a concise and structured format that are invaluable for last minute revision. During clinical years, it will be ideal for brushing up on basic concepts.

We would like to thank Elliott Smock for allowing us this opportunity. It would not have been possible without the exceptional help and guidance from Professor Milligan. Thank you to everyone who has supported us – you know who you are!

We wish you the very best for your exams and your future careers!

ABBREVIATIONS

ACE	angiotensin-converting enzyme		ICSI	intracytoplasmic sperm injection
ACTH	adrenocorticotrophic hormone		IGFs	insulin-like growth factors
ADH	antidiuretic hormone/vasopressin		IgG	immunoglobulin G
AMH	anti-mullerian hormone		IgM	immunoglobulin M
ASD	atrial septal defect		IUD	intrauterine device
ATP	adenosine triphosphate		IVF	*in vitro* fertilization
BMI	body mass index		IVC	inferior vena cava
BMR	basal metabolic rate		K^+	potassium
CNS	central nervous system		LDL	low-density lipoprotein
Ca^{2+}	calcium		LH	luteinizing hormone
cAMP	cyclic adenosine monophosphate		MAO A + B	monoamine oxidase A + B
CBG	cortisol-binding globulin		MIT	monoiodotyrosine
CCK	cholecystokinin		mRNA	messenger ribonucleic acid
cGMP	cyclic guanosine monophosphate		MS	multiple sclerosis
CMV	cytomegalovirus		MSH	melanocyte-stimulating hormone
CNS	central nervous system		OGTT	oral glucose tolerance test
COCP	combined oral contraceptive pill		OTC	oxytocin
COMT	catecholmethyltransferase		PDA	patent ductus arteriosus
CRH	corticotrophin-releasing hormone		PIF	prolactin-inhibiting factor
DA	dopamine		PMS	premenstrual syndrome
DHEA	dehydroepiandrosterone		POP	progestogen-only pill
DIT	diiodotyrosine		PPi	inorganic pyrophosphate
DM	diabetes mellitus		PRL	prolactin
DNA	deoxyribonucleic acid		PS	pulmonary stenosis
FSH	follicle-stimulating hormone		PTU	propylthiouracil
GFR	glomerular filtration rate		PTH	parathyroid hormone
GH	growth hormone		Rh	rhesus
GHIH	growth hormone-inhibiting hormone		SHBG	sex hormone-binding globulin
GHRH	growth hormone-releasing hormone		SIADH	syndrome of inappropriate ADH secretion
GI	gastrointestinal			
GIP	gastric inhibitory peptide		SRY	sex-determining region on the Y chromosome
GnRH	gonadotrophin-releasing hormone			
hCG	human chorionic gonadotrophin		SS	somatostatin
HDL	high-density lipoprotein		SV	stroke volume
HIV	human immunodeficiency virus		T3	triiodothyronine
hPL	human placental lactogen		T4	thyroxine
HR	heart rate		TAG	triglyceride
HRT	hormone replacement therapy		TBG	thyroxine-binding globulin

TBPA	thyroxine-binding pre-albumin	VDR	vitamin D receptor
TRH	thyrotrophim-releasing hormone	VMA	vanilmandelic acid
TSH	thyroid-stimulating hormone	VSD	ventricular septal defect

SECTION 1

ENDOCRINE SYSTEMS AND THE HYPOTHALAMIC–PITUITARY AXIS

ENDOCRINE SYSTEMS AND THE HYPOTHALAMIC–PITUITARY AXIS

1. Is it true or false that hormones

a. Are always released from glands
b. Are secreted via ducts
c. Act via specific receptors
d. Are secreted into the bloodstream
e. Are always released in response to neural stimuli

2. Regarding hormones

a. The brain is an endocrine organ
b. The gastrointestinal tract is not an endocrine organ
c. The pancreas secretes glucagon
d. The thyroid gland secretes calcitonin
e. The posterior pituitary synthesizes antidiuretic hormone and oxytocin

3. Regarding the endocrine system

a. Endocrine dysfunction always results in hormone deficiency
b. Pituitary adenoma causes hypofunction of the pituitary gland
c. Primary endocrine dysfunction can occur at the level of the thyroid
d. An inability of the cells to produce hormone results in hyposecretion
e. Graves' disease is an example of hyposecretion

4. Give three characteristics of a hormone

GI, gastrointestinal; T4, thyroxine

EXPLANATION: ENDOCRINE SYSTEMS AND THEIR IMPORTANCE IN DISEASE

A **hormone** is a chemical substance released from a **ductless** gland (or group of secretory cells) **directly into the bloodstream** in response to a **stimulus** and exerts a **specific regulatory effect** on its **target organ(s) via receptors (4)**. The main **endocrine** organs of the body are as follows:

Organ		Hormones secreted	Abbreviation
Brain	Hypothalamus	Somatostatin	SS
		Corticotrophin-releasing hormone	CRH
		Growth hormone-releasing hormone	GHRH
		Gonadotrophin-releasing hormone	GnRH
		Thyrotrophin-releasing hormone	TRH
		Dopamine	DA
	Pituitary (anterior)	Adrenocorticotrophic hormone	ACTH
		Growth hormone	GH
		Follicle-stimulating hormone	FSH
		Luteinizing hormone	LH
		Thyroid-stimulating hormone; Prolactin	TSH; PRL
	Pituitary (posterior)	Antidiuretic hormone and oxytocin	ADH
Thyroid		Thyroxine	T4
		Calcitonin	
GI tract		Gastrin	
		Cholecystokinin	CCK
		Gastrointestinal peptide	
		Secretin	
Pancreas		Insulin; Glucagon; Somatostatin; Pancreatic polypettide	
Adrenals		Cortisol; Aldosterone	
Ovaries and testes		Testosterone; Oestradiol; Progesterone	

Endocrine dysfunction can occur at different levels, for example, at the level of hormone production and secretion (e.g. failure to produce a hormone), or at the level of the target organ (e.g. failure to respond to a hormone due to lack of receptors). It can be classified into hyper- and hyposecretion. Hypersecretion can be due to a tumour that secretes **excess hormone** (e.g. pituitary adenoma) or due to an **inappropriate stimulation** (e.g. in Graves' disease antibodies stimulate the thyroid to produce excess T4). Hyposecretion can be due to the **inability** of cells to produce hormone (e.g. in hypothyroidism there is a reduction in the amount of T4 secreted) or due to **hypofunction** of a gland (e.g. excess **somatostatin** release from the **hypothalamus** results in a decrease in the amount of **growth hormone** released by the anterior pituitary).

Answers

1. F F T T F
2. T F T T F
3. F F T T F
4. See explanation

5. In clinical endocrinology

a. Measurement of steroid levels in saliva gives a reflection of plasma hormone levels
b. Measurement of steroid levels in urine gives a reflection of secretion over the previous several hours
c. Bioassay is the measurement of the biological responses induced by a hormone
d. Immunoassays are both sensitive and specific
e. Immunoassays detect the level of hormone antigen in the plasma

6. Draw a diagram that illustrates the integration of the nervous and hormonal control systems in the body

7. Briefly outline the concept of feedback control

EXPLANATION: BASIC PRINCIPLES OF CLINICAL ENDOCRINOLOGY

The **endocrine system** is controlled by **positive and negative feedback**. Positive feedback acts to **stimulate release** of hormones; negative feedback acts to **inhibit release** of hormones **(7)**.

The integration of nervous and hormonal control systems in the body is illustrated below **(6)**.

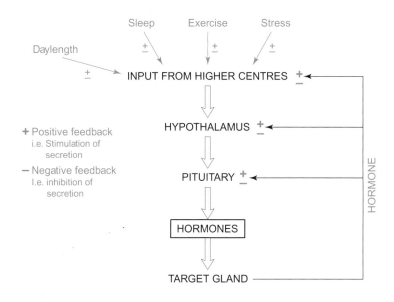

Hormones are present in low concentrations in the circulation and **bind to receptors** in target cells with **high affinity and specificity**.

Hormone levels in urine and plasma samples can be estimated using:

- **Bioassays** – measurement of **biological responses** induced by the hormone
- **Immunoassays** – measurement of the amount of hormone present by using **antibodies** that are raised to bind to specific antigenic sites on the hormone. They are **sensitive and precise**. Their specificity depends on the specificity of the antibody.

NB: the measurement of **steroid hormone** levels in the urine represents a reflection of secretion over the previous several hours.

Answers

5. T T T T T
6. See explanation
7. See explanation

8. With regard to steroid hormones

a. Thyroid-stimulating hormone is an example
b. They bind to a receptor in the cytoplasm or nucleus
c. They exert their effects via a second messenger mediated system
d. They affect the rate of transcription of specific genes
e. They are secreted from the smooth endoplasmic reticulum

9. Concerning peptide hormones

a. Insulin is an example
b. They bind to receptors in the cell nucleus
c. They are water soluble
d. They are secreted from the rough endoplasmic reticulum
e. They stimulate protein synthesis through activation of second messengers

10. Draw a table comparing peptide hormone secretory cells with steroid hormone secretory cells

11. Outline the mechanism by which a hormone causes an intracellular response via a second messenger

ADH, antidiuretic hormone; GH, growth hormone; TSH, thyroid-stimulating hormone; FSH, follicle-stimulating hormone; T4, thyroxine; cAMP, cyclic adenosine monophosphate; cGMP, cyclic guanosine monophosphate

EXPLANATION: MICROSTRUCTURE OF THE ENDOCRINE SYSTEM

Hormones can be:

- Amino acid derivatives, e.g. adrenaline
- Small peptides, e.g. vasopressin (ADH)
- Proteins, e.g. GH, insulin
- Glycoproteins, e.g. TSH, FSH
- Steroids, e.g. cortisol, oestradiol
- Tyrosine derivatives, e.g. noradrenaline, T4.

The secretory cells that produce different types of hormone have distinct ultrastructural characteristics (10).

Peptide/protein hormone-secreting cells	Steroid hormone-secreting cells
Large rough endoplasmic reticulum Large Golgi apparatus Secretory vesicles	Large smooth endoplasmic reticulum Many lipid vacuoles

Steroid hormones (e.g. sex hormones, adrenal corticosteroids, vitamin D) are lipophilic (**water insoluble**) and often circulate in the blood **bound** to **proteins**. When they enter cells they combine with highly specific **receptor** proteins in the **cytoplasm** or **nucleus**. The hormone–receptor complex then **acts within the cell nucleus**, where it binds to hormone response elements on the **nuclear DNA**, promoting the synthesis of specific **proteins**. These then mediate the effects of the hormones.

Protein and polypeptide hormones (e.g. glucagon, insulin) are water soluble and circulate largely in free form. They do not penetrate into the cell interior but react with receptors located in the **cell membrane**. This can result in **direct membrane** effects or **intracellular** effects mediated by **second messenger systems** (e.g. cAMP, cGMP, protein kinase C) within the cell (11).

The actions of water-soluble and -insoluble hormones are compared in the diagrams given on page 24.

12. Name three gastrointestinal hormones and state their roles

13. Match the following hormones of the gastrointestinal system with the statements below

Options

    A. Cholecystokinin
    B. Secretin
    C. Gastrin
    D. Gastric inhibitory peptide

    1. It is secreted by G-cells in the stomach
    2. Its release is stimulated by acidic pH
    3. It enhances insulin secretion
    4. It stimulates contraction of the gall bladder
    5. It stimulates the release of hydrochloric acid from the parietal cells

14. Regarding gastrointestinal hormones

    a. All gastrointestinal hormones are secreted from the duodenum
    b. The presence of fat stimulates release of both cholecystokinin and gastric inhibitory peptide
    c. A pH of 8 would stimulate release of secretin
    d. Gastric inhibitory peptide is secreted from G-cells
    e. The breakdown products of proteins stimulate release of gastrin

GI, gastrointestinal; CCK, cholecystokinin; GIP, gastric inhibitory peptide; HCl, hydrochloric acid; $HCO_3{}^-$, bicarbonate

EXPLANATION: GASTROINTESTINAL HORMONES

The **GI hormones** are produced by '**clear**' cells, so-called because they appear under the microscope to have a clear cytoplasm with a large nucleus. These are distributed **diffusely** throughout the gut. The GI hormones and their roles are listed below (12).

Hormone	Site of synthesis	Stimulus for release	Action
Gastrin	**G-cells**, which are located in gastric pits, primarily in the antrum region of the **stomach**	Presence of **peptides** and **amino acids** in the gastric lumen	Release of **HCl** from **parietal cells** of the stomach. Regulates growth of gastric mucosa
CCK	Mucosal **epithelial cells** in the first part of the **duodenum**	Presence of **fatty acids** and **amino acids** in the small intestine	Contraction of the **gall bladder** Stimulates release of pancreatic enzymes
GIP	Mucosal **epithelial cells** in the first part of the **duodenum**	Presence of **fat** and **glucose** in the small intestine	**Enhances insulin secretion** from the pancreatic islet cells under conditions of hyperglycaemia
Secretin	Mucosal **epithelial cells** in the first part of the **duodenum**	**Acidic pH** in the lumen of the small intestine	Stimulate HCO_3^- **secretion** from the pancreas Potentiates **CCK**-invoked release of pancreatic enzymes

Answers

12. See explanation
13. 1 – C, 2 – B, 3 – D, 4 – A, 5 – C
14. F T F F T

15. Match the following hormones of the hypothalamic–pituitary axis with the statements below

Options

A. Growth hormone-releasing hormone
B. Somatostatin
C. Dopamine
D. Thyrotrophin-releasing hormone
E. Gonadotrophin-releasing hormone
F. Corticotrophin-releasing hormone

1. Stimulates release of follicle-stimulating hormone
2. Inhibits release of growth hormone
3. Stimulates release of growth hormone
4. Stimulates release of prolactin
5. Stimulates release of adrenocorticotrophic hormone

16. Briefly describe how a challenge test can be used to investigate the function of an endocrine system

17. Regarding hormones

a. The hypothalamus is derived from the diencephalon
b. The anterior pituitary is derived from the primordial oral cavity
c. Rathke's pouch is derived from the endoderm
d. Pituicytes are found in the anterior pituitary
e. The adenohypophysis contains hormone-secreting cells

GH, growth hormone; TRH, thyrotrophin-releasing hormone; TSH, thyroid-stimulating hormone; PRL, prolactin; ACTH, adrenocorticotrophic hormone; GnRH, gonadotropin-releasing hormone; CRH, corticotropin-releasing hormone; GHRH, growth hormone-releasing hormone; PIF, prolactin-inhibiting factor; LH, luteinizing hormone

EXPLANATION: HYPOTHALAMUS AND PITUITARY

Embryologically, the **hypothalamus** is derived from the **diencephalon**. The **anterior pituitary** (adenohypophysis) is derived from Rathke's pouch, which is an ectodermal pouch of the primordial oral cavity. The **posterior pituitary** (neurohypophysis) is an extension of the nervous system.

Features of the microscopic structure of pituitary gland are:

- Adenohypophysis: vascular sinusoids, hormone-secreting cells and connective tissue
- Neurohypophysis: fibrous material consisting of axons and neuroglial cells (pituicytes).

Hypothalamic releasing or inhibiting factors are listed below.

Releasing or inhibiting factor	Abbreviation	Function
GH-releasing hormone	GHRH	Stimulates release of GH
Somatostatin	SS	Inhibits release of GH
Prolactin-inhibiting factor (dopamine)	PIF	Inhibits release of PRL
Thyrotrophin-releasing hormone	TRH	Stimulates release of TSH and PRL
Gonadotrophin-releasing hormone	GnRH	Stimulates release of LH and FSH
Corticotrophin-releasing hormone	CRH	Stimulates release of ACTH

TESTS OF FUNCTION

Challenge tests are used to **investigate how a system is working** and where it is going wrong, i.e. is it a problem at the hypothalamic/pituitary or some other level. For example, **provocative tests** of pituitary function are based on using a known stimulus to **see if the system can respond**. For example, administration of TRH normally results in increased TSH and PRL at 30 minutes, with levels declining at 60 minutes. **Suppression tests** are used to **see if the normal feedback mechanisms are operating** or whether something is **over-riding** them. For example, oral administration of glucose normally suppresses GH release, although subsequently there is enhancement as blood sugar falls. In acromegalic patients, release of GH is not suppressed, so the excessive secretion of GH continues **(16)**.

Answers

15. 1 – E, 2 – B, 3 – A, 4 – D, 5 – F
16. See explanation
17. T T F F T

18. Complete the table below, linking the correct site of synthesis with the correct hormone. The first one has been done for you

Hormone	Site of synthesis
GH	Somatotrophs
PRL	1
TSH	2
ACTH	3
FSH	4
LH	5

19. Pituitary hormones (e.g. ACTH) can be released in a diurnal pattern. Give two examples of other patterns of pituitary hormone release. Which hormones follow these patterns?

20. Write a short paragraph on the control of the anterior pituitary. Include the following points: pituitary portal vessels, hypothalamus, stimulation or inhibition

GH, growth hormone; PRL, prolactin; TSH, thyroid-stimulating hormone; ACTH, adrenocorticotrophic hormone; FSH, follicle-stimulating hormone; LH, luteinizing hormone; ADH, antidiuretic hormone

EXPLANATION: ANTERIOR PITUITARY

The **anterior pituitary** consists of cuboidal/polygonal epithelial secretory cells clustered around large fenestrated sinusoids which enable efficient transport of hormone into the blood.

The anterior pituitary hormones are listed below.

Hormone	Site of synthesis
GH	Somatotrophs
PRL	Mammotrophs
TSH	Thyrotrophs
ACTH	Corticotrophs
FSH	Gonadotrophs
LH	Gonadotrophs

There are three main patterns of pituitary hormone release **(19)**:

- **Circadian/diurnal** – most hormones, including ACTH, PRL, ADH (vasopressin)
- **Infradian/pulsatile** (variations superimposed on circadian changes) – e.g. ACTH, GH, LH
- **Longer term variations** (e.g. over menstrual cycle) – e.g. FSH and LH (female); many hormones show age-related changes.

CONTROL OF ANTERIOR PITUITARY

Neuroendocrine cells of the **hypothalamus** whose **axons** project to the **median eminence** regulate the anterior pituitary. They **secrete hormones** into the capillaries of the **pituitary portal vessels**, which in turn end in capillaries bathing the cells of the anterior pituitary. The hypothalamic hormones either stimulate or inhibit the release of hormones from the anterior pituitary **(20)**.

Answers

18. 1 – mammotrophs; 2 – thyrotrophs; 3 – corticotrophs; 4 – gonadotrophs; 5 – gonadotrophs
19. See explanation
20. See explanation

21. Fill in the table below – the first row has been done for you

Trophic hormone	Stimulus for release	Target organ	Action on target organ	Regulation
TSH	TRH	Thyroid follicle	Production of thyroxine	Feedback inhibition by rising thyroxine levels
ACTH				
MSH				
FSH				
LH				
GH				
PRL				

22. Match the following hormones with the statements below

Options

A. Adrenocorticotophic hormone
B. Prolactin
C. Thyroid-stimulating hormone
D. Follicle-stimulating hormone
E. Luteinizing hormone
F. Growth hormone
G. Melanocyte-stimulating hormone

1. Stimulates the bone, muscle, adipose tissue and the liver
2. Is inhibited by rising thyroxine levels
3. Stimulates spermatogenesis
4. Stimulates the mammary glands
5. Stimulates the production of cortisol

23. Draw a diagram showing the control of prolactin secretion

TSH, thyroid-stimulating hormone; TRH, thyrotrophin-releasing hormone; MSH, melanocyte-stimulating hormone; FSH, follicle-stimulating hormone; CRH, corticotrophin-releasing hormone; LH, luteinizing hormone; GnRH, gonadotrophin-releasing hormone; GHRH, growth hormone-releasing hormone; ACTH, adenocorticotrophic hormone; GH, growth hormone; PRL, prolactin; IGFs, insulin-like growth factors

EXPLANATION: PITUITARY HORMONES

The table below summarizes the release and action of the pituitary hormones (21).

Trophic hormone	Stimulus for release	Target organ	Action on target organ	Regulation
TSH	TRH	Thyroid follicle	Production of thyroxine	Feedback inhibition by rising thyroxine levels
ACTH	CRH	Adrenal cortex	Production of cortisol	Feedback inhibition by rising cortisol levels
MSH	MSH-releasing factor UV light exposure ACTH	Melanocytes	Pigmentation	MSH-inhibiting factor
FSH	GnRH	Ovary Testis	Follicle growth, oestrogen production Spermatogenesis	Feedback control by gonadal steroids
LH	GnRH	Ovary Testis	Follicle growth, ovulation, luteal function Production of testosterone, spermatogenesis	Feedback control by gonadal steroids
GH	GHRH; inhibited by somatostatin	Muscle Bone Adipose tissue Liver	Stimulation of cell growth and expansion Antagonizes the actions of insulin	Feedback control by IGFs
PRL	TRH; inhibited by dopamine	Mammary glands	Stimulation of development of mammary glands and milk secretion	

The diagram illustrates the control of prolactin secretion (23).

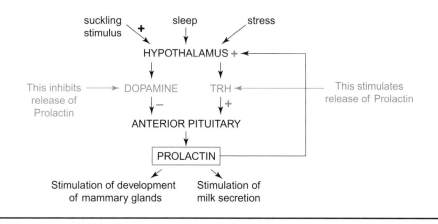

Answers
21. See explanation
22. 1 – F, 2 – C, 3 – D, 4 – B, 5 – A
23. See explanation

24. The following are features of Syndrome of Inappropriate ADH secretion (SIADH)

a. Excess antidiuretic hormone
b. Renal failure
c. Retention of water
d. High plasma osmolality
e. Normal adrenal function

25. Diabetes insipidus

a. Is characterized by production of large volumes of dilute urine
b. Is never caused by head injury
c. Diagnosis is made by the dexamethasone suppression test
d. Is due to excess vasopressin secretion
e. Can be caused by damage to the neurohypophyseal system

26. The following inhibit release of ADH

a. Rise in temperature
b. Nausea and vomiting
c. Reduced plasma osmolality
d. Negative feedback on hypothalamic osmoreceptors
e. Pain

27. Oxytocin release is stimulated by

a. Suckling
b. Parturition
c. Stress
d. Rise in progesterone
e. Vaginal distension

ADH, antidiuretic hormone; SIADH, syndrome of inappropriate ADH secretion

EXPLANATION: POSTERIOR PITUITARY

The **posterior pituitary** consists of **axons** of modified neurons, supported by a group of glial-like cells called **pituicytes**. The cell bodies of these neurons lie in the **supraoptic** and **paraventricular** nuclei of the hypothalamus.

Two hormones are released by the posterior pituitary: **ADH (vasopressin)** and **oxytocin**.

ADH

ADH release is stimulated by an **increase in osmotic pressure** in the circulating blood; haemorrhage; pain and trauma; nausea and vomiting; rise in temperature. It causes **retention of water by the kidney**, which **reduces plasma osmolality**. It acts on the final section of the distal convoluted tubule and on the collecting ducts to increase their permeability to **water** and therefore its **reabsorption**. It also raises blood pressure by contracting vascular smooth muscle cells.

ADH is regulated through **reduced** plasma **osmolality** acting as a **negative feedback** signal on the hypothalamic osmoreceptors, which suppress ADH secretion.

SIADH is a condition characterized by **hypersecretion of ADH**. The result is retention of water, low plasma osmolality, **concentrated urine**, normal renal and adrenal function. Causes can include brain trauma and infection, pneumonia and malignant disease, and cytotoxic therapy. Treatment is to **restrict fluid intake**.

In **diabetes insipidus** large volumes of **dilute urine** are produced due to a reduction in or absence of **ADH secretion**. It is most commonly caused by damage to the neurohypophyseal system, for example, as the result of head injury or growth of a tumour. A **water-deprivation test** may be used to confirm the diagnosis: the body is **unable to concentrate the urine**, so the flow of urine continues and the patient loses weight.

OXYTOCIN

Oxytocin release is stimulated by **vaginal stimulation** at parturition and **nipple stimulation** during suckling. It acts by contracting smooth muscle cells, especially of the uterus during childbirth and myoepithelial cells of the mammary gland during lactation.

A **positive-feedback** mechanism operates to regulate oxytocin release during childbirth when the fetus stretches the cervix. Oxytocin causes muscle contraction, causing increased stretching, which stimulates further release of oxytocin. Suckling also stimulates oxytocin secretion, but stress inhibits the release of oxytocin and so reduces the flow of milk.

Answers
24. T F T F T
25. T F F F T
26. F F T T F
27. T T F F T

28. GH release is stimulated by

a. Sleep
b. Stress
c. Hypoglycaemia
d. Exercise
e. Growth hormone-releasing hormone

29. GH deficiency leads to

a. Increase in body fat
b. Hypertension
c. Hyperinsulinaemia
d. Glucose intolerance
e. Decreased muscle strength

30. The following are characteristics of acromegaly

a. Excess growth hormone
b. Joint pain
c. Increase in body fat
d. Hypertension
e. Lethargy and fatigue

31. Draw a diagram showing the control of release of GH

32. Outline the effects of GH on carbohydrates, proteins, lipids and IGFs

Disorders associated with GH deficiency or excess production include:

Hyposecretion (GH deficiency)	Hypersecretion (GH excess) (Acromegaly)
In children – short and fat with characteristic facies	Lethargy or fatigue
Loss of growth rate	Joint pain
Increase in body fat and decreased muscle strength	Hyperinsulinaemia
(due to loss of metabolic functions of GH)	Glucose intolerance
	Hypertension
	Soft tissue overgrowth
	Enlargement of heart

GH, growth hormone; GHRH, GH-releasing hormone; IGFs, insulin-like growth factors; ACTH, adrenocorticotrophic hormone

EXPLANATION: GROWTH

The diagram below shows the mechanisms underlying the regulation of GH **(31)**.

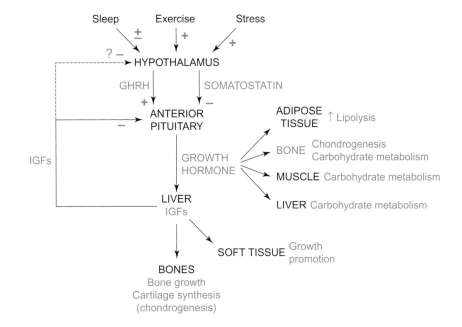

GH secretion is stimulated by both physiological and pharmacological factors:

- **Physiological** – exercise, stress, sleep and post-prandial glucose decline
- **Pharmacological** – hypoglycaemia, amino acid infusions, small peptide hormones (e.g. ACTH), monoaminergic stimuli and non-peptide hormones.

The actions of GH on various substrates are as follows **(32)**:

- **Carbohydrates** – GH increases blood glucose, decreases peripheral insulin sensitivity (is diabetogenic), increases hepatic output of glucose
- **Proteins** – GH increases tissue amino acid uptake, increases amino acid incorporation into protein, decreases urea production and nitrogen balance
- **Lipids** – GH is lipolytic, and after long administration can be ketogenic, particularly in diabetics
- **IGFs** – GH stimulates production of IGFs from the liver and other tissues. They mediate GH's growth-related effects. A number of disorders are associated with a deficiency or excess production of GH.

See opposite for a table of disorders associated with GH deficiency or excess production.

Answers
28. T T T T T
29. T F F F T
30. T T F T T
31. See explanation
32. See explanation

33. Draw a diagram illustrating the diurnal variation in GH secretion

34. Regarding circadian rhythms

    a. Growth hormone secretion is solely influenced by circadian rhythms
    b. The hypothalamus is involved in control of circadian rhythms
    c. The supraoptic nucleus acts as a clock by providing timing cues
    d. Melatonin secretion is maximal at night
    e. Body temperature is affected by circadian rhythms

35. Answer true or false to the following

    a. Testosterone secretion is maximal at night
    b. Testosterone secretion decreases with increasing age
    c. Retinal ganglion cells are involved in detecting changes in environmental light
    d. Urine output is not affected by circadian rhythms
    e. Growth hormone secretion is maximal at midday

EXPLANATION: CIRCADIAN RHYTHMS

A **circadian rhythm** describes the regular recurrence, in cycles of **about 24 hours**, of biological processes, such as hormone secretion, sleeping, feeding, etc. This rhythm seems to be regulated by a '**biological clock**' that is set by recurring daylight and darkness. In mammals, the biological clock lies in the individual neurons of the **suprachiasmatic nucleus** in the hypothalamus.

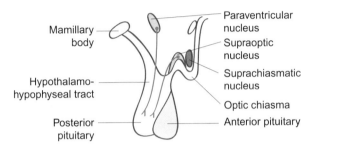

The suprachiasmatic nucleus receives signals from the environment and provides **timing cues**. Circadian rhythms are co-ordinated by 'clock genes' whose protein products reflect different phases of the daily cycle.

Circadian rhythms are seen in most physiological parameters (e.g. sleep/wake cycle, body temperature, urine output). The clock in the **suprachiasmatic nucleus** also controls the **pineal secretion** of melatonin. **Melatonin** secretion is maximal at night and probably helps to co-ordinate circadian rhythmicity, although the mechanism is unclear. The exact mechanism of detecting changes in environmental light is also unclear. Among the theories suggested, melanopsin, which is found in the retinal ganglion cells, has been proposed.

A number of systems are affected by a light/dark (sleep/wake) cycle, for example, core body temperature and melatonin secretion from the pineal gland.

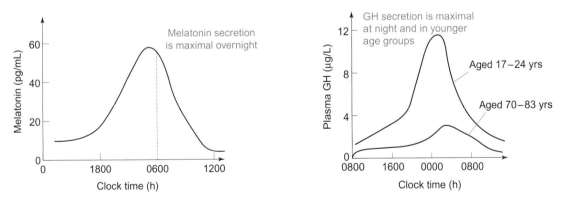

In addition to **variation** with a **light/dark cycle**, there are also **age-related changes** in endocrine function. **GH** is secreted at **increased** levels at night, but this level is dramatically **reduced** with **increasing age**. In contrast, **testosterone** secretion is **decreased** with **increasing age**.

Answers
33. See diagram
34. F T F T T
35. F T T F F

36. Leptin

    a. Is a steroid hormone
    b. Is secreted by adipose tissue
    c. Receptors are found in both the ovaries and the hypothalamus
    d. Promotes a signal reflecting the energy state of the body
    e. Is solely involved in the control of appetite

37. Consider leptin

    a. Leptin release is stimulated by a high body mass index
    b. Leptin acts to inhibit insulin
    c. Both catecholamines and androgens inhibit release of leptin
    d. Long-term hyperinsulinaemia stimulates release of leptin
    e. Leptin stimulates appetite

38. Draw a diagram showing the actions of leptin and the factors that affect its secretion

BMI, body mass index; CNS, central nervous system

EXPLANATION: ADIPOSE TISSUE

Leptin is a **protein hormone** that is secreted by white **adipose (fat) tissue**. Leptin receptors have been found in the hypothalamus, pancreas, ovaries, testes, uterus, kidneys, heart, lungs and skeletal tissue. Leptin provides a **signal** reflecting the **energy states** of the body and may be involved in the control of appetite and reproduction. It **reduces food intake** and **increases energy expenditure**. Obese people tend to have high leptin levels.

The actions of leptin and the factors that affect its secretion are illustrated below.

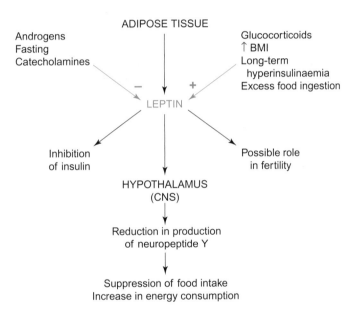

MICROSTRUCTURE OF THE ENDOCRINE SYSTEM: continued from page 7.

The actions of water-soluble and -insoluble hormones are compared in the diagrams below.

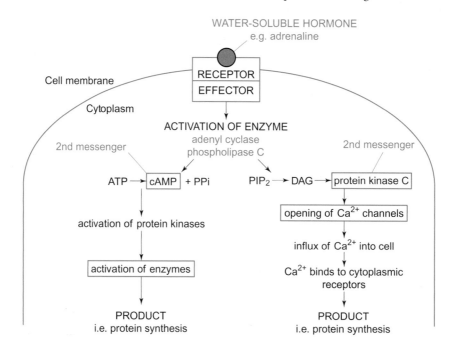

This process activates pre-existing protein enzymes

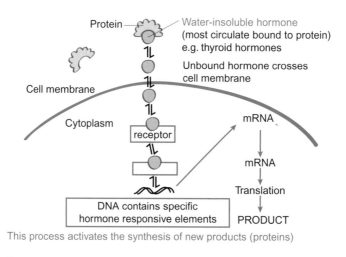

This process activates the synthesis of new products (proteins)

ATP, adenosine triphosphate; PPi, inorganic pyrophosphate; DAG, diacylglycerol; mRNA, messenger RNA; DNA, deoxyribonucleic acid

THYROID AND PARATHYROIDS

2 THYROID AND PARATHYROIDS

1. Outline the congenital malformations of the thyroid that may result from abnormal development

2. Name the anatomical relations, the blood supply, and the venous and lymphatic drainage of the thyroid gland

3. In the thyroid and parathyroid glands

    a. Thyroglobulin accumulates in follicles as colloid
    b. Calcitonin is secreted by thyroid follicles
    c. Parafollicular cells originate in the neural crest
    d. Parathyroid hormone is secreted from principal cells
    e. The thyroid develops from the endodermal floor of the pharyngeal cavity

EXPLANATION: ANATOMY

The adult thyroid gland weighs 10–20 g. It is nearly always asymmetric and it is usually larger in women than it is in men.

Anatomical relations of thyroid and parathyroid glands are shown in the diagram (2):

Thyroid development commences at day 24 as a **midline thickening** and then as an outpouching of the **endodermal floor** of the pharyngeal cavity, which then descends. The **parathyroid glands** are derived from the epithelium of the **third and fourth pharyngeal pouches**.

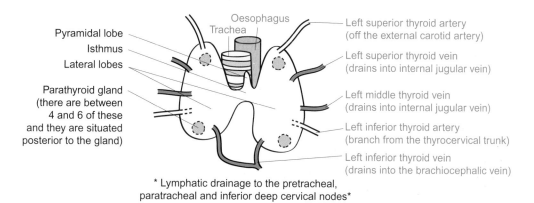

Pyramidal lobe
Isthmus
Lateral lobes

Parathyroid gland
(there are between
4 and 6 of these
and they are situated
posterior to the gland)

Oesophagus
Trachea

Left superior thyroid artery
(off the external carotid artery)

Left superior thyroid vein
(drains into internal jugular vein)

Left middle thyroid vein
(drains into internal jugular vein)

Left inferior thyroid artery
(branch from the thyrocervical trunk)

Left inferior thyroid vein
(drains into the brachiocephalic vein)

* Lymphatic drainage to the pretracheal,
paratracheal and inferior deep cervical nodes*

Congenital abnormalities of the thyroid and parathyroid include (1):

- Persistent thyroglossal duct
- Failure of thyroid to descend to correct level, resulting in a thyroid gland in the sublingual or intrathoracic positions
- Development of only a single thyroid lobe
- Complete absence of thyroid – very rare, but serious as it can lead to the development of **cretinism**.

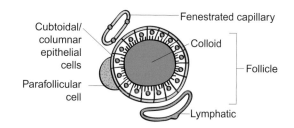

Cubtoidal/
columnar
epithelial
cells

Parafollicular
cell

Fenestrated capillary

Colloid

Follicle

Lymphatic

On the microscopic level, thyroid epithelial cells are organized into **follicles** that secrete **thyroglobulin** (which accumulates in follicles as colloid). The **C-cells (parafollicular cells) secrete calcitonin** and are found within the follicular epithelium or as clusters between the follicles. They are larger and more rounded than the follicle cells and originate from the neural crest in the embryo.

The **parathyroid glands** consist of densely packed, small **chief cells** (principal cells) arranged in irregular cords around blood vessels, which secrete **parathyroid hormone** (parathormone).

Answers
1. See explanation
2. See explanation
3. T F T T T

4. Regarding triiodothyronine and tyroxine

    a. Only triiodothyronine is cleaved from thyroglobulin
    b. Triiodothyronine and thyroxine are bound to plasma proteins
    c. Thyroxine contains three molecules of iodine
    d. Thyroid hydroxylase is the main enzyme involved in thyroid hormone synthesis
    e. Thyroxine is excreted in the bile

5. What are the key steps in the synthesis of triiodothyronine and tyroxine

6. Draw a diagram of the feedback loop regulating thyroid hormone secretion

7. Thyroid-stimulating hormone

    a. Acts on the thyroid follicles
    b. Stimulates iodination of thyroglobulin
    c. Stimulates release of triiodothyronine only
    d. Is released by the hypothalamus
    e. Is regulated by thyroxine

T3, triiodothyronine; T4, thyroxine; TSH, thyroid-stimulating hormone; TRH, thyrotrophin-releasing hormone; MIT, monoiodotyrosine; DIT, diiodotyrosine; TBG, thyroxine-binding globulin; TBPA, thyroxine-binding pre-albumin

EXPLANATION: T3 AND T4

TSH is secreted by the anterior pituitary gland. It acts on the thyroid follicles stimulating **colloid** droplets, which contain **thyroglobulin**, to be taken up into the thyroid cell cytoplasm. Following lysosomal fusion and proteolysis, **T3 and T4** are cleaved from thyroglobulin.

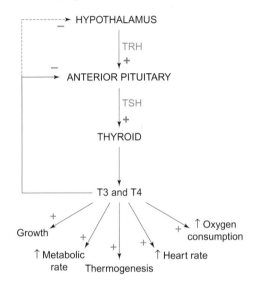

Synthesis of T3 and T4 involves active uptake of **iodine** from the blood by the thyroid follicular cells and incorporation of iodine atoms into **tyrosol** residues of thyroglobulin (5). The addition of iodine to tyrosol residues of thyroglobulin is catalysed by **thyroid peroxidase** to give MIT and DIT. The combination of MIT + DIT gives T3 and DIT + DIT gives T4. T3 and T4 are cleaved from thyroglobulin as required.

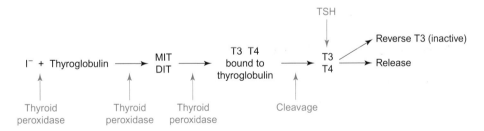

In plasma, T3 and T4 are **strongly bound to serum proteins**, such as TBG, TBPA and serum albumin, restricting their access to cells and their potential biological activity. Only 0.015 per cent of T4 and 0.33 per cent of total serum T3 are present in the **free/active** form. Stores and plasma levels of **protein-bound** T4 are 20 times those of T3. T4 is excreted in the bile following a process of deiodination.

Answers
4. F T F F T
5. See explanation
6. See diagram
7. T T F F T

8. List the four main actions of thyroid hormones

9. Thyroid hormones

    a. Are vital for growth and development
    b. Act to increase basal metabolic rate
    c. Are produced in equal quantities
    d. Increase heart rate
    e. Are secreted in increased amounts in cold temperatures

10. Thyroid hormones

    a. Stimulate mRNA production
    b. Bind to extracellular receptors
    c. Act via nuclear receptors
    d. Increase the number of adrenoreceptors
    e. Decrease adenosine triphosphate turnover

T3, triiodothyronine; T4, thyroxine; ATP, adenosine triphosphate; BMR, basal metabolic rate; TRH, thyrotrophin-releasing hormone; CNS, central nervous system; mRNA, messenger ribonucleic acid; TSH, thyroid-stimulating hormone

EXPLANATION: THYROID HORMONES

T4 has a half-life of 7 days; T3 of 1 day. **T3** is the main **biologically active hormone**, although more T4 is secreted. T4 is converted to T3 in peripheral tissues by deiodinase enzymes.

Thyroid hormones bind to **intracellular receptors** that are similar to **steroid receptors** (i.e. stimulate mRNA production). They act to increase Na^+/K^+ ATPase levels (and thus increase ATP turnover), increase O_2 consumption, **increase BMR** and increase the number of adrenoreceptors.

The main physiological actions of the thyroid hormones are as follows (8):

1. **Calorigenesis**: T3 and T4 increase the rate of O_2 consumption by the heart, skeletal muscle, liver and kidney. In adults, brain, spleen and gonad metabolism is less susceptible to the effects of T3 and T4. In cold conditions, CNS input through the hypothalamus (TRH) increases TSH, and T3 and T4 secretion to **increase metabolic rate**, thus maintaining body temperature.
2. **Carbohydrate and fat metabolism** is increased.
3. **Growth and development** regulation, especially in the fetus. T3 and T4 impact upon numerous systems, including muscle, bone, CNS development, myelination, dendritic formation and synapse formation.
4. **Cardiovascular**: T4 and T3 have cardiovascular effects, increasing the heart rate and force of contraction to achieve **increased cardiac output**. In hyperthyroidism, the number of beta-adrenergic receptors in the heart is increased (beta-adrenergic receptor antagonists are sometimes used as part of treatment).

Answers
8. See explanation
9. T T F T T
10. T F T T F

11. List three causes of hypothyroidism, giving the origin of the dysfunction

12. Explain the term goitrogen and give two examples

13. Match the following thyroid disorders with the statements below

Options

A. Hashimoto's thyroiditis
B. Pituitary tumour
C. Cretinism
D. Graves' disease
E. Toxic nodular goitre
F. Thyroiditis

1. Is a benign neoplasm
2. Destroys thyroid tissue
3. Is an autoimmune disorder
4. Is secondary hypofunction of the thyroid
5. Is a congenital disorder

TSH, thyroid-stimulating hormone; TRH, thyrotrophin-releasing hormone; T3, triiodothyronine; T4, thyroxine

EXPLANATION: THYROID DYSFUNCTION

The causes of hypofunction of the thyroid (**hypothyroidism**) are as follows (**11**):

- **Primary**, e.g. Hashimoto's thyroiditis (chronic immune disease) – insufficient synthesis of thyroid receptors due to **destruction of thyroid tissue** in thyroiditis; **cretinism** (congenital lack of thyroid tissue); radiotherapy for hyperthyroidism (which destroys thyroid cells); iodine deficiency (iodine requirement = 150 μg/day)
- **Secondary**, e.g. Pituitary tumours
- **Tertiary**, e.g. Hypothalamic lesion.

Hyperfunction of the thyroid (**hyperthyroidism**) is caused by:

- **Graves' disease** (diffuse toxic goitre) – the thyroid becomes enlarged and produces too much thyroid hormone due to stimulation by antibodies (see page 35)
- **Toxic nodular goitre** (benign neoplasm) – the cells in the nodule produce **excess** thyroid hormone
- **Thyroiditis** (inflammation of the thyroid).

A **goitrogen suppresses thyroid hormone production**, resulting in increased TSH production and enlargement of the thyroid gland (goitre) due to compensatory stimulation of thyroid follicles. Goitrogenic substances include kelp (high doses of iodine), cabbage and cassava (glycosides), lithium and some cough mixtures (**12**).

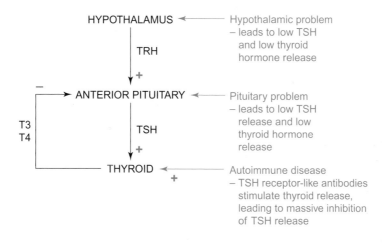

Answers

11. See explanation
12. See explanation
13. 1 – E, 2 – A, 3 – D, 4 – B, 5 – C

14. Explain how autoantibodies may mimic a stimulating hormone, giving a clinical example

15. Give three features associated with Graves' disease

16. What is the physiological basis of the symptoms seen in thyroid disease?

17. Complete the table below with the symptoms of hypo- and hyperthyroidism. The first row has been done for you

Clinical symptoms	Hyperthyroidism	Hypothyroidism
Appearance	Weight loss, sweating, tremor, goitre	Weight gain, coarse skin, dry hair, hoarse voice, puffy appearance
Disposition		
Cardiac function		
Neuromuscular function		
Others		

18. In Graves' disease

   a. There is hypertrophy of thyroid follicular cells
   b. There is decreased synthesis of thyroid hormones
   c. There is a low thyroid-stimulating hormone level
   d. There is a goitre
   e. There is thyrotoxicosis

TSH, thyroid-stimulating hormone; T4, thyroxine; BMR, basal metabolic rate; IgG, immunoglobulin G

EXPLANATION: SYMPTOMS OF THYROID DYSFUNCTION

The effects of **hypothyroidism** in adults are the result of a **lowered metabolic rate**. Conversely, many of the classic symptoms of **hyperthyroidism** are due to an **increased basal metabolic rate** and **enhanced beta-adrenergic activity** (16). NB: TSH and T4 influence the BMR; the BMR does not affect them, although temperature does.

The following table lists the symptoms of hyperthyroidism and hypothyroidism (myxoedema) (17).

Clinical symptoms	Hyperthyroidism	Hypothyroidism
Appearance	Weight loss, sweating, tremor, maybe a goitre	Weight gain, coarse skin, dry hair, hoarse voice, puffy appearance
Disposition	Agitated and nervous, easy fatiguability, heat intolerance	Cold, particularly at extremities, lethargic, depressed
Cardiac function	Tachycardia and atrial fibrillation	Reduced cardiac output, so slow pulse
Neuromuscular function	Muscle weakness and loss of muscle mass	Generalized muscle weakness and paraesthesiae; slow relaxing tendon reflexes
Others	Diarrhoea, shortness of breath, infertility, amenorrhoea; rapid growth rate and accelerated bone maturation in children	Menstrual irregularities

The most common cause of hyperthyroidism is Graves' disease: This is an **autoimmune disease**. Antibodies (called thyroid-stimulating antibodies) of the IgG1 subclass bind to TSH receptors on the thyroid follicular cell membrane causing **stimulation of adenylate cyclase**. This results in hypertrophy of the follicular cells, increased synthesis and secretion of thyroid hormones, and **goitre** formation (14). This is a clear example of how autoantibodies can mimic a stimulating hormone. There is a **high circulating T4** concentration due to the increased stimulation, and a **low TSH** concentration due to negative feedback on the hypothalamic–pituitary axis.

Features associated with Graves' disease include the following (15):

- **Triad of goitre, eye signs and thyrotoxicosis (hyperthyroidism)** – eye signs include upper lid retraction, stare, periorbital oedema, redness and swelling of the conjunctiva, exophthalmos, impaired eye movement, inflammation of cornea
- Pretibial myxoedema – thickening of skin over the lower tibia due to deposition of glycosaminoglycans
- Others – vitiligo, acropachy (clubbing of fingertips), proximal myopathy, fine tremor.

Answers

14. See explanation
15. See explanation
16. See explanation
17. See explanation
18. T F T T T

19. What is the treatment for hyperthyroidism?

20. Describe the mechanisms of action of propylthiouracil?

21. In thyroid disease

- **a.** Iodine supplementation is used to treat hyperthyroidism
- **b.** Radioiodine is used to treat hyperthyroidism
- **c.** Beta-blockers block the parasympathetic effects of thyroid hormones
- **d.** Thyroxine administration can be used in treatments of both hyper- and hypothyroidism
- **e.** Surgery is always used to treat hyperthyroidism

T4, thyroxine; PTU, propylthiouracil; T3, triiodothyronine

EXPLANATION: TREATMENT OF THYROID DISEASE

Hyperthyroidism is treated using antithyroid drugs, either a **block-replacement regimen**, using a high dose of an antithyroid drug, such as **carbimazole** or **propylthiouracil**, together with T4 replacement, or **beta-blockers**, for example, propanolol (blocks the sympathetic effects of thyroid hormones). Alternatively, it can be treated with **radioiodine** ('kills' thyroid cells) or **surgically** (subtotal ablation of the gland) **(19)**.

PTU **inhibits iodine and peroxidase** from interacting normally with thyroglobulin to form T4 and T3. This action decreases thyroid hormone production. It also interferes with the conversion of T4 to T3, and, since T3 is more potent than T4, this also reduces the activity of thyroid hormones **(20)**.

Hypothyroidism is treated through thyroid hormone replacement with oral T4 or liothyronine (Na^+ salt of T3), or with iodine supplementation.

Answers

19. See explanation
20. See explanation
21. F T F T F

22. **Explain the importance of the parathyroid glands**

23. **In the regulation of calcium**

    a. Ca^{2+} absorption is increased by diets containing brown bread
    b. Ca^{2+} absorption is increased by diets containing milk
    c. The majority of the body's Ca^{2+} is stored in the bone
    d. Ca^{2+} exists bound to plasma proteins as well as its free ionic form
    e. The reference value for plasma Ca^{2+} is 500 mM

24. **Calcium is involved with**

    a. Hormone release
    b. Muscle contraction
    c. Cardiac muscle
    d. Neuromuscular junction excitability
    e. Bone mineral formation

25. **Outline the relationship between phosphate and calcium**

PTH, parathyroid hormone

EXPLANATION: FUNCTION OF PARATHYROID GLANDS

Parathyroid glands produce **PTH** (parathormone) which is important in Ca^{2+} and PO_4^{3-} homeostasis (22).

There is a total of about 1 kg of Ca^{2+} in the adult body, and about 99 per cent of it is in bone, in the form of **hydroxyapatite**. An **equilibrium** is reached between **absorption** and **excretion**. Ca^{2+} levels within the body are closely associated with those of PO_4^{3-} and they work together to carry out the following functions (25):

- **Bone** formation and maintenance
- **Muscle contraction** including cardiac muscle
- All processes that involve exocytosis, including synaptic transmission and hormone release.

Normal Ca^{2+} and PO_4^{3-} levels are as follows:

- Plasma Ca^{2+} 2.5 mM (2.2–2.6 mM)
- Free ionic form of Ca^{2+} 1.2 mM
- Ca^{2+} bound to plasma proteins   1 mM
- Ca^{2+} complex, e.g. with citrate   0.3 mM
- Plasma PO_4^{3-} 0.8–1.4 mmol

Factors that affect absorption of Ca^{2+} are listed in the following table.

Increase absorption	Decrease absorption
Dietary lactose	Fibre
Basic amino acids, e.g. high protein, milk	Phytic acid, e.g. in fortification of brown bread
Vitamin D from sunlight and diet	Increasing age
Children, pregnancy, lactation	

Answers

22. See explanation
23. F T T T F
24. T T T T T
25. See explanation

26. Give two signs of hypercalcaemia

27. Outline the mechanism of action of parathyroid hormone on bone

28. Match the following calcium-regulating substances with the statements below

Options

    A. Parathyroid hormone
    B. Cholecalciferol
    C. Calcitonin

    1. Increases plasma PO_4^{3-}
    2. Is secreted when plasma Ca^{2+} is high
    3. Binds to intracellular receptors
    4. Increases Ca^{2+} reabsorption in the kidney
    5. Binds to receptors on bone-forming cells

PTH, parathyroid hormone; cAMP, cyclic adenosine monophosphate; VDR, vitamin D receptor; mRNA, messenger ribonucleic acid; ATP, adenosine triphosphate; DNA, deoxyribonucleic acid

EXPLANATION: REGULATION OF CALCIUM

The effects of **PTH**, **calcitonin** and **vitamin D** on Ca^{2+} levels are listed in the following table.

	Plasma Ca^{2+}	Plasma PO_4^{3-}
PTH	↑	↓
Vitamin D (cholecalciferol)	↑	↑
Calcitonin	↓	↓

PTH acts on **bone** by binding with receptors on **osteoblasts** (bone-forming cells), causing an increase in cAMP and inhibiting collagen synthesis. These cells then release soluble factors such as **prostaglandins** and **interleukin**, which cause osteoclasts to release their Ca^{2+} and PO_4^{3-} content. There is also increased osteoclast collegenase activity and therefore increased osteolytic activity, which results in **increasing plasma Ca^{2+} levels** (27).

In the **kidney**, PTH causes **increased Ca^{2+} reabsorption** in the distal tubule and decreased PO_4^{3-} reabsorption in the proximal and distal tubules, resulting in **increased PO_4^{3-}** excretion. It also activates 1 alpha-hydroxylase, which is needed for the conversion of vitamin D into its active form.

Calcitonin is secreted from **C-cells** (parafollicular cells) when plasma Ca^{2+} is high. It acts on **osteoclasts** via cAMP and **suppresses** their activity. NB: Osteoclasts are involved in bone demineralization.

Vitamin D is produced in the skin from 7-dehydrocholesterol by UV radiation. The liver and other tissues metabolize vitamin D by 25-hydroxylation to 25-OH-D, the principal circulating form of vitamin D. 25-OHD is then further metabolized to $1,25(OH)_2D$ in the kidney: this is the principal hormonal form of vitamin D, responsible for most of its biologic actions. Vitamin D has genomic and non-genomic actions:

- Genomic – vitamin D acts as a **steroid hormone** and binds to an **intracellular receptor** (VDR) in the intestinal mucosal cell. The VDR binds DNA and promotes synthesis of mRNA and proteins, many of which are **Ca^{2+}-binding proteins** (calbindins). These have a great affinity for Ca^{2+} at the brush border membrane of the intestinal mucosa and they facilitate transport of Ca^{2+} to the basolateral membrane, thus **increasing plasma Ca^{2+}** levels. They also activate the Ca^{2+} ATPase pump at the basolateral side, which pumps Ca^{2+} out of the cell into the plasma.
- Non-genomic – vitamin D has a **direct** effect on cell membranes causing rapid stimulation of **Ca^{2+} transport** (transcaltachia) via the opening of voltage-gated Ca^{2+} channels, and activation of a vesicular mechanism of Ca^{2+} transport involving microtubules and calbindin.

Common signs of hypo- and hypercalcaemia are listed in the table below.

Hypocalcaemia	Hypercalcaemia (26)
Hyperexcitable nervous system	Nervous response sluggish
Tetany	Ectopic calcification (kidneys, synovial membrane)
Plasma Ca^{2+} <1.5 mM = lethal	Plasma Ca^{2+} >3.75 mM = lethal

Answers

26. See explanation
27. See explanation
28. 1 – B, 2 – C, 3 – B, 4 – A, 5 – A

29. Lack of calcium absorption from the gut can result in osteomalacia or rickets – list the characteristics of these

30. Groups at risk of osteomalacia include

   a. Breast-fed babies
   b. Elderly people
   c. Women of Asian origin
   d. Lactating mothers
   e. Housebound people

31. Match the following calcium-related disorders with the statements below

Options

   A. Vitamin D-resistant rickets
   B. Osteomalacia
   C. Rickets

   1. A cause is phenytoin therapy
   2. A cause is lack of Ca^{2+} absorption in the gut in adults
   3. Is characterized by bone pain
   4. Is characterized by decreased mineral:matrix ratio in children
   5. Results from defective 25-hydroxylation

EXPLANATION: OSTEOMALACIA AND RICKETS

Osteomalacia occurs in adults and rickets in children as a result of a **lack of Ca²⁺ absorption** from the **gut**. In both, there is a decrease in the mineral:matrix ratio of bone.

Groups at risk of osteomalacia and rickets include:

- Breast-fed babies
- Children and women of Asian origin, especially those on vegetarian diets low in Ca^{2+} and high in phytate
- Elderly and housebound people.

Osteomalacia is characterized by **bone pain**, increased incidence of bone fractures and 'thin' bones on X-ray, and other features of hypocalcaemia.

There are two types of **rickets (29)**:

1. Rickets due to **vitamin D deficiency** – the characteristics of which are '**knock-knees**' or '**bow-legs**' caused by bending of long bones, postural abnormalities and other features of hypocalcaemia
2. Vitamin D-resistant rickets – this may be due to **defective 25-hydroxylation** because of liver disease or defective enzyme production; or **defective 1-hydroxylation** because of renal disease or defective enzyme production. Other causes include **barbiturate** and **phenytoin** therapy (for epilepsy), chronic renal failure and a mutation on the X-chromosome that causes an X-linked disorder.

Answers

29. See explanation
30. T T T F T
31. 1 – A, 2 – B, 3 – B, 4 – C, 5 – A

SECTION 3

ADRENALS AND PANCREAS

ADRENALS AND PANCREAS

1. Give the anatomical relations of the adrenal gland

2. Match the following parts of the adrenal glands with the statements below

Options

    A. Cortex
    B. Medulla

    1. It is the innermost part of the adrenal gland
    2. It is derived from the neural crest
    3. It consists of three zones
    4. Its cells secrete adrenaline
    5. Its cells secrete steroids

3. Draw a diagram of the microstructure of the adrenal gland

EXPLANATION: ADRENAL GLANDS

The cells of the adrenal **cortex** are organized into three zones: zona glomerulosa, zona fasciculata and zona reticularis. These secrete **steroids**. The **medulla** consists of large cells arranged in clumps or cords that receive a stimulatory cholinergic input. On stimulation, they secrete **catecholamines** (adrenaline and noradrenaline). The cells of the **medulla** stain when treated with chromate salts due to the reaction with catacholamines and are often referred to as **chromaffin** cells.

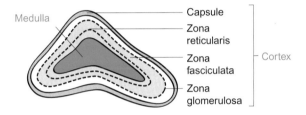

The anatomical relations of the adrenal glands are shown in the table below **(1)**.

Left		Right
Anterior	Splenic vessels + pancreas	Vena cava + right lobe of liver
Posterior	Left crus of diaphragm	Right crus of diaphragm
Inferior	Upper pole of left kidney	Upper pole of right kidney
Superior	Stomach	

- Blood supply: Derived from a circle of arteries arising from the superior, middle and inferior arteries – capsular vessels, cortical vessels and medullary arterioles
- Nerve supply: Splanchnic nerves
- Venous and lymphatic drainage: The central vein of the right adrenal drains into the inferior vena cava, while on the left, it drains into the left renal vein.

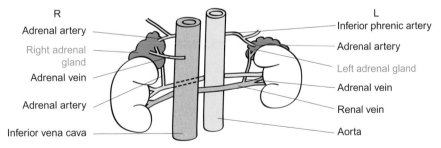

DEVELOPMENT OF THE ADRENAL GLANDS

The **cortex** is derived from the epithelium (mesothelium) lining the embryonic coelomic cavity. The **medulla** is derived from the **neural crest** and is a modified sympathetic ganglion.

Answers

1. See explanation
2. 1 – B, 2 – B, 3 – A, 4 – B, 5 – A
3. See diagram

4. Name the three zones of the adrenal cortex and give examples of their secretions

5. Match the following substances with the statements below

Options

A. Cortisol
B. Aldosterone
C. Adrenaline
D. Corticotrophin-releasing hormone
E. Adrenocorticotrophic hormone
F. Dehydroepiandrosterone

1. Is stimulated by the renin–angiotensin pathway
2. Is released by the hypothalamus
3. Stimulates the adrenal cortex to produce steroids
4. Potentiates the synthesis of catecholamines
5. Is an adrenal androgen

ACTH, adrenocorticotrophic hormone; DHEA, dehydroepiandrosterone; cAMP, cyclic adenosine monophosphate; CRH, corticotrophin-releasing hormone

EXPLANATION: ADRENAL CORTEX

The **adrenal cortex** is under the control of **ACTH**. The **zona fasciculata** produces **glucocorticoids** (e.g. cortisol); the **zona glomerulosa** produces **mineralocorticoids** (e.g. aldosterone) and the **zona reticularis** produces **adrenal androgens** (e.g. DHEA) **(4)**. All **steroids** are synthesized from **cholesterol**.

ACTH binds to high-affinity adrenal receptors on the adrenal cortical cell, increasing intracellular concentrations of cAMP. This enhances transport of cholesterol and activation of cholesterol ester hydroxylase, resulting in increased production of steroids.

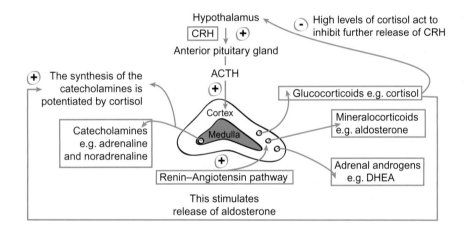

6. Name two enzymes involved in steroid biosynthesis from cholesterol, and state which steps they are involved in

7. Draw the basic chemical structure of steroids

8. Put the following steps of biosynthesis of steroids into the correct order:

   A. Further transformation of pregnenolone
   B. Side-chain cleavage to produce pregnenolone
   C. Transportation of cholesterol from storage droplets into the mitochondria
   D. Hydrolysis of cholesterol esters
   E. Transport of pregnenolone out of the mitochondria into smooth endoplasmic reticulum

9. Regarding hormones

   a. Cortisol and oestrogen are cholesterol derivatives
   b. A deficiency in adrenocorticotrophic hormone leads to feminization of newborn males
   c. The C-ring structure of steroids has no bearing on the physiological action of steroids
   d. Steroid hormones are synthesized and secreted as required
   e. Pregnenolone is synthesized in the mitochondria

EXPLANATION: STEROIDOGENESIS

All steroids are derived from **cholesterol** and share a **characteristic chemical structure** that accounts for the physiological action of steroids. Cholesterol is made up of **three hexagonal carbon rings** (A, B, C) and a **pentagonal carbon ring** (D) to which a side chain (carbons 20–27) is attached. Two angular methyl groups are also found at position 18 and 19.

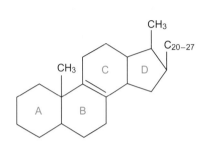

Changes to the side chain give rise to different compounds. These individual compounds are characterized by the presence or absence of specific **functional groups** (mainly hydroxy, keto(oxo) and aldehyde functions for the naturally occurring steroids) at certain positions of the carbon skeleton.

Steroid hormones are not stored but are synthesized and secreted as required.

Deficiencies of the **enzymes** involved in steroidogenesis can occur with resulting hormone imbalance:

- 21-Hydroxylase deficiency (this accounts for 95 per cent of all cases)
- Congenital virilizing adrenal hyperplasia
- Congenital 17 alpha-hydroxylase deficiency
- Congenital lipoid adrenal hyperplasia
- Corticosterone methyl oxidase (type II) deficiency.

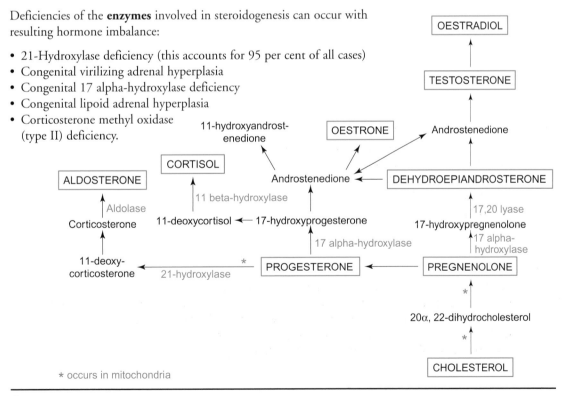

* occurs in mitochondria

Answers

6. See diagram
7. See diagram
8. 1 – D, 2 – C, 3 – B, 4 – E, 5 – A
9. T F F T T

10. In glucocortoid disease

a. A diabetes test should be performed in a patient presenting with symptoms of Cushing's syndrome

b. Cushing's syndrome is caused by cortisol deficiency

c. Cortisol deficiency can lead to hyperkalaemia

d. Centripetal obesity and striae are characteristics of Cushing's syndrome

e. There is increased pigmentation of skin in Addison's disease

11. Give three causes of hypersecretion of glucocorticoids

12. Give five symptoms of Cushing's syndrome

13. Cortisol

a. Is a glucocorticoid

b. Controls the effects of adrenaline

c. Adapts the body's response to stress

d. Is secreted maximally at night

e. Circulates bound to cortisol-binding globulin

14. Addison's disease

a. Results from increased plasma levels of cortisol

b. Is characterized by increased adrenocorticotrophic hormone release

c. Causes hypertension

d. Causes hypokalaemia

e. Can occur as a result of the treatment of inflammatory disorders

ACTH, adrenocorticotrophic hormone; CBG, cortisol-binding globulin

EXPLANATION: GLUCOCORTICOIDS

Cortisol is the major **glucocorticoid**. It circulates bound to CBG and has three main physiological actions:

1. It maintains the responsiveness of target cells to adrenaline and noradrenaline
2. It maintains metabolic balance
3. It adapts the body's **response** to **stress** by preventing it from over-responding (e.g. suppresses inflammation).

There is a **circadian (diurnal) rhythm** to plasma cortisol levels, although it is probably secreted all the time in varying amounts. Levels are **higher** in the morning and **lower** at night.

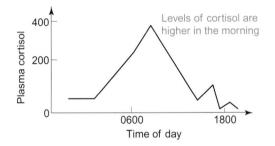

Hypersecretion of glucocorticoids can be caused by pituitary adenoma, adrenal adenoma or carcinoma, and ectopic ACTH syndrome **(11)**. NB: **High plasma levels** can also be caused by excess administerd glucocorticoids. It results in increased lipolysis and fat redeposition, increased protein breakdown, increased liver glucose production and aldosterone-like effects.

Cortisol excess results in **Cushing's syndrome**, characterized by **(12)**:

- Round 'moon' face
- Striae
- Muscle wasting/weakness
- Infections
- **Diabetes**
- Buffalo hump
- Truncal obesity
- **Bruising**
- **Hypertension**
- Osteoporosis.

Hyposecretion of glucocorticoids can result from exogenous steroids causing feedback inhibition, for example, prednisolone given to suppress inflammatory or allergic disorders; and surgical removal of ACTH-producing tumours. It causes reduced lipolysis, reduced protein breakdown, a tendency to salt and water depletion, and a tendency to hypercalcaemia.

Cortisol deficiency results in secondary Addison's, the symptoms of which include:

- Increased pigmentation of skin and mucosa caused by increased ACTH release
- Lethargy
- Hyperkalaemia
- Postural hypotension.

NB: **Addison's disease** can be due to either a primary cause, where there is lack of both cortisol and aldosterone (as seen in chronic insufficiency of the adrenal cortex, e.g. caused by autoimmune disease and TB infection) or a secondary cause where there is lack of cortisol only (e.g. in pituitary ACTH deficiency).

Answers
10. T F T T T
11. See explanation
12. See explanation
13. T T T F T
14. F T F F T

15. Draw a diagram outlining the renin–angiotensin–aldosterone pathway

16. Outline the features of Conn's syndrome

17. In mineralocorticoid disorders

    a. Conn's syndrome occurs when there is hypersecretion of aldosterone
    b. A decrease in plasma K^+ stimulates release of aldosterone
    c. Aldosterone acts to promote Na^+ reabsorption
    d. Changes in blood Na^+ activate the renin–angiotensin–aldosterone pathway
    e. Changes in blood osmolality stimulate antidiuretic hormone secretion

18. Match the following with the statements below

Options

    A. Aldosterone   **B.** Angiotensin II
    C. Antidiuretic hormone   **D.** Renin
    E. Adrenocorticotrophic hormone

    1. Decreases the rate of Na^+ secretion
    2. Is stimulated by changes in blood Na^+
    3. Is stimulated by changes in blood osmolality
    4. Increases the rate of K^+ excretion
    5. Is released by the anterior pituitary gland

19. Hyposecretion of aldosterone

    a. Can be caused by tuberculosis
    b. Causes hypotension
    c. Causes high plasma K^+ levels
    d. Results in hypertension
    e. Is caused by adrenal adenoma

ACTH, adrenocorticotrophic hormone; ADH, antidiuretic hormone

EXPLANATION: MINERALOCORTICOIDS

Aldosterone is a major **mineralocorticoid**. It circulates bound to plasma albumin. It acts directly on the kidney to:

- decrease the rate of Na^+ excretion (with accompanying retention of water)
- increase the rate of K^+ excretion.

Stimuli for aldosterone secretion include **angiotensin II**, **increased plasma K^+** concentration and **ACTH**. It is controlled by the pathways shown below.

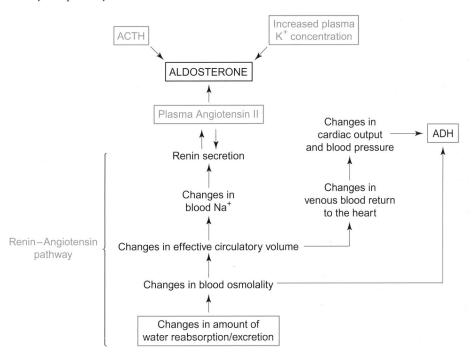

Hypersecretion of aldosterone (**Conn's syndrome**) is caused by adrenal adenoma, where tumour cells secrete excess aldosterone, and adrenal hyperplasia. It results in hypokalaemia, hypokalaemia alkalosis and **hypertension (16)**.

Hyposecretion of aldosterone (**primary Addison's syndrome**) is caused by **autoimmune disease**, **tuberculosis**, and **malignancy**. Its symptoms include **hyperkalaemia**, mild metabolic acidosis and hypotension.

Answers

15. See diagram
16. See explanation
17. T F T T T
18. 1 – A, 2 – D, 3 – C, 4 – A, 5 – E
19. T T T F F

20. Outline the pathway for the synthesis of adrenaline and noradrenaline

21. Regarding hormones of the adrenal medulla

   a. Noradrenaline is a tyrosine derivative
   b. Both noradrenaline and adrenaline are degraded to vanilmandelic acid
   c. Adrenaline mediates the stress response 'fight or flight'
   d. Noradrenaline only affects the systolic blood pressure
   e. Adrenaline causes pupillary constriction

22. Concerning hormones

   a. Phaeochromocytoma results in hypertension
   b. Adrenomedullary hyposecretion has severe clinical consequences
   c. Adrenal atrophy results in adrenomedullary hypersecretion
   d. Hypertension is seen in adrenomedullary hypersecretion
   e. Pallor, headaches and sweating are associated with excess adrenaline release

MAO, monoamine oxidase; COMT, catechomethyltransferase; VMA, vanilmandelic acid

EXPLANATION: ADRENAL MEDULLA

The synthesis and degradation of the **catecholamines** are shown below **(20)**.

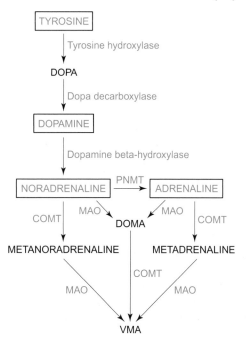

Adrenaline release is stimulated by **stress** (e.g. exercise, pain, fear, hypotension, hypoglycaemia, hypoxia). The effects of adrenaline include increased systolic blood pressure, but reduced diastolic blood pressure, tachycardia, reduced gut motility, bronchodilatation, piloerection and **dilatation of pupils**. It also promotes hepatic glycogenolysis, leading to hyperglycaemia and lactic-acidaemia. Adrenaline is regulated via the hypothalamic–pituitary–adrenal axis and degradation is via MAO A and B and COMT to VMA.

Noradrenaline release is also stimulated by **stress** (e.g. exercise, pain, fear, hypotension, hypoglycaemia, hypoxia). It has the effect of raising both systolic and diastolic blood pressure, so increasing mean blood pressure. It also causes bradycardia, piloerection, dilatation of pupils, and mobilization of free fatty acids. Regulation is via the hypothalamic–pituitary–adrenal axis and degradation is via MAO A and B and COMT to VMA.

Adrenomedullary hypersecretion is caused by phaeochromocytoma (catecholamine-secreting tumour), resulting in hypertension, neuroblastomas and ganglioneuromas. It results in **hypertension,** pallor, headaches, sweating and glucose intolerance.

Adrenomedullary hyposecretion is caused by adrenal atrophy. There are **no clinical consequences** due to compensation for catecholamine deficiency by the nervous system.

Answers
20. See explanation
21. T T T F F
22. T F F T T

23. Name the anatomical relations of the pancreas

24. Match the following cell types of the endocrine pancreas to their secretions

Options

A. Alpha cells
B. Beta cells
C. Delta cells
D. F or PP cells

1. Secrete insulin
2. Secrete somatostatin
3. Secrete glucagon
4. Secrete pancreatic polypeptide

25. Regarding the pancreas

a. The pancreas is derived from the midgut
b. The acinar cells release bicarbonate via the pancreatic duct
c. The pancreas is a retroperitoneal organ
d. The islets of Langerhans are exocrine cells
e. The B cells secrete insulin

HCO_3^-, bicarbonate

EXPLANATION: PANCREAS

The **pancreas** is a retroperitoneal organ. It consists of a head with an uncinate process, a neck, a body and a tail. Embryologically, it arises from dorsal and ventral endodermal outgrowths from the foregut, which then form a branching duct system.

The anatomical relations of the pancreas are as follows (23):

• Head: Lies within curve of the duodenum, in front of the vena cava
• Tail: Reaches hilus of spleen.

Blood is supplied to the pancreas by branches of the **splenic artery**, and **superior** and **inferior pancreatico-duodenal arteries**. Nerve supply is from the splanchnic nerves and the vagi via the coeliac plexus, and lymphatic drainage is to the coeliac group of pre-aortic nodes via the suprapancreatic nodes.

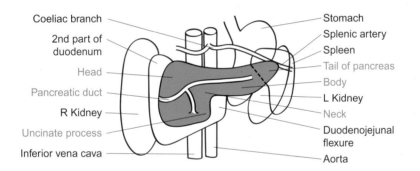

The **exocrine** cells (acinar cells) of the pancreas release digestive enzymes and HCO_3^- into the duodenum via the pancreatic duct. The **endocrine** cells (islets of Langerhans) are small, rounded clusters of cells embedded within the exocrine pancreas. The cells are smaller and more lightly stained than the exocrine cells, and are arranged in irregular cords around the capillaries. Four main cells types can be distinguished using immunocytochemistry (24):

• A or alpha cells which secrete **glucagon**
• B or beta cells which secrete **insulin**
• D or delta cells which secrete **somatostatin**
• F or PP cells which secrete **pancreatic polypeptide**.

Answers
23. See diagram and explanation
24. 1 – B, 2 – C, 3 – A, 4 – D
25. F T T F T

26. Increased secretion of the following occurs in the fasting state:

    a. Adrenaline
    b. Glucagon
    c. Insulin
    d. Glucocorticoids
    e. Noradrenaline

27. Briefly outline the effect on blood glucose level of the release of insulin and glucagon

28. Give an example of a cause of hyperglycaemia and the resulting clinical characteristics

29. The following can be seen in hypoglycaemia

    a. Tachycardia
    b. Vomiting
    c. Hyperventilation
    d. Boils on the skin
    e. Impaired consciousness

GH, growth hormone; DM, diabetes mellitus

EXPLANATION: GLUCOSE HOMEOSTASIS

Glucose is the **principal energy source for tissues of the body**, and uptake by many peripheral tissues requires a minimal, though continuous, secretion of insulin. When blood glucose levels are high, **insulin** is released. When blood glucose levels are low, **glucagon** is released **(27)**. Because of the dual and opposite actions of insulin and glucagon, hypoglycaemia does not develop in the fasting state or during exercise. In addition, **adrenaline, cortisol and GH** are involved in the **regulation** of **plasma glucose levels**.

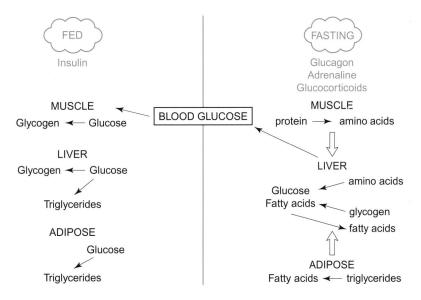

Hyperglycaemia is caused by **diabetes mellitus** as a result of impaired insulin secretion and/or insulin resistance by the tissues, or, very rarely, by glucagonoma **(28)**. It has the following effects:

- **Glycosuria**
- Salt and water depletion
- Weight loss due to protein degradation to supply glucose
- Vomiting

- Tiredness and weakness
- Tachycardia, hypotension and hyperventilation
- Infections (pruritus vulvae and boils)
- Impaired consciousness and visual acuity
- Convulsions and coma (if severe).

Hypoglycaemia occurs as a complication of the treatment of DM (insulin overdose plus insufficient carbohydrate intake), during fasting in a patient with a non-diabetic disorder and can occur as **postprandial hypoglycaemia** after a meal. It causes **adrenergic symptoms** (e.g. sweating, tachycardia and tremor) due to increased catacholamine release, and **neuroglycopenic symptoms** (e.g. blurred vision, slurring of speech, unsteadiness of gait and impaired consciousness) due to deficiency of glucose supply to the brain.

Answers
26. T T F T F
27. See explanation
28. See explanation
29. T F F F T

30. Type 2 diabetes mellitus

    a. Usually presents with ketoacidosis
    b. Has a late onset
    c. Can be due to insulin resistance in the tissues
    d. Has no genetic basis
    e. Cannot be controlled by diet only

31. With regard to type 1 diabetes mellitus

    a. It has a juvenile onset
    b. Islet cell antibodies are only present in 20 per cent of cases
    c. Insulin therapy is required
    d. It is caused by a total/near total insulin deficiency
    e. There is a positive family history in 60 per cent of cases

32. The following are not seen in type 2 diabetes mellitus

    a. Hyperventilation
    b. Polydipsia
    c. Polyuria
    d. Weight loss
    e. Islet cell antibodies

33. Give five features associated with type 1 diabetes mellitus

34. Give an example where overproduction of another hormone can give rise to the clinical syndrome of diabetes mellitus

growth hormone - acromegaly

DM, diabetes mellitus; GH, growth hormone

EXPLANATION: DIABETES MELLITUS

Type 1 DM usually has a **juvenile onset** and is caused by total or near-total **insulin deficiency**. This results from the destruction of **beta cells** in the pancreas. Islet cell antibodies are present in 85 per cent of cases. The cause of the **autoimmune** disease is usually idiopathic but can be secondary to viral infections of the pancreas and toxins. There is also a strong genetic component (e.g. 50 per cent concordance in identical twins and a positive family history in 10 per cent of patients). Patients require **insulin therapy**.

Type 2 DM has a late onset and is often associated with **obesity**. It is caused by **impaired insulin secretion** from the pancreas, and/or **insulin resistance** in the tissues (there is a post-receptor defect so it is the signalling pathway inside the cell that is affected). There is almost a 100 per cent concordance in identical twins and a positive family history in 30 per cent of patients. Patients are advised to **lose weight** and watch their **diet**. Those not controlled by diet need to take **oral hypoglycaemia agents** to increase the secretion of insulin or potentiate its actions. In the advanced stages of disease, insulin may be required.

The following table compares the features of type 1 and type 2 DM.

Features exclusive to type 1 (33)	Features common to type 1 and 2	Features exclusive to type 2
Ketones on breath	Tiredness, impaired consciousness, impaired visual acuity	
Hyperventilation	Polydipsia, vomiting	
Weight loss prior to presentation	Tachycardia, hypotension	Minimal weight loss
Ketonuria (ketones in the urine)	Muscle weakness and wasting	No or trace of ketonuria
+/− ketoacidosis	Polyuria and prone to kidney infections	Not associated with ketoacidosis, although ketosis can occur
Islet cell antibodies present	Prone to skin infections, e.g. pruritus vulvae and boils	Islet cell antibodies not present

Overproduction of some hormones can give rise to the clinical syndrome of DM as their actions oppose insulin, for example, in acromegalic patients where the elevated GH acts against insulin (34).

Answers

30. F T T F F
31. T F T T F
32. T F F T T
33. See explanation
34. See explanation

35. **Give three lifestyle changes that can be made in the management of type 2 diabetes mellitus**

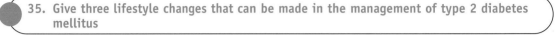

- exercise
- diet restriction
- less alcohol (?), no smoking

36. **State four aims of therapy in diabetes mellitus**

37. **Match the following diagnoses with the fasting plasma glucose levels below**

Options

A. Normal
B. Diabetes mellitus
C. Impaired fasting glycaemia/impaired glucose tolerance

1. 9 mmol/L fasting venous plasma glucose
2. 14 mmol/L OGTT venous plasma glucose
3. 4 mmol/L fasting venous plasma glucose
4. 6.5 mmol/L fasting venous plasma glucose
5. 4.5 mmol/L OGTT venous plasma glucose

EXPLANATION: DIAGNOSIS AND MANAGEMENT OF DIABETES MELLITUS

The **diagnosis** of DM requires a **fasting venous plasma glucose level over 7.0 mmol/L** in the **presence of symptoms** of DM (such as polyuria and polydipsia). The normal level is <6.1 mmol/L. A level of 6.0–7.0 implies there is either impaired fasting glycaemia or impaired glucose tolerance.

If the fasting venous plasma glucose is >7 mmol/L but there are no symptoms, an **OGTT** must be performed. A level of **>11.1 mmol/L** is diagnostic (OGTT is an oral glucose tolerance test where a glucose load is given and blood glucose level is measured after 2 hours).

A full examination of the patient must always be performed to exclude signs of complications.

Management of DM aims to (36):

- Minimize **hypoglycaemia**
- Relieve **symptoms** and prevent long-term complications
- Provide **education and support**, and improve quality of life, for example, introduce to a specialist nurse, dietician and chiropodist.

Lifestyle changes have an important role in the management of type 2 DM. They include the adoption of a **diet** that is high in carbohydrate and low in fat and refined sugars, stopping **smoking**, and taking adequate **exercise**. Home glucose monitoring is recommended (35).

Answers

35. See explanation
36. See explanation
37. 1 – B, 2 – B, 3 – A, 4 – C, 5 – A

38. Match the following with the statements below

Options

3 **A.** Alpha-glucosidase inhibitors 5 11 **B.** Biguanides

7 **C.** Sulphonylureas **D.** Thiazolidinediones

1. Increase glucose uptake
2. Increase insulin release
3. Prevent the post-prandial increase in glucose
4. Decrease insulin resistance
5. Metformin is an example

39. Write short notes on the use of insulin to treat type 1 diabetes mellitus

40. Concerning insulin therapy

F **a.** Insulin can be given orally

F **b.** Infection reduces insulin requirements

F **c.** Insulin reduces glucose uptake

F **d.** All patients receive identical insulin regimens

T **e.** Type 1 diabetes mellitus patients always require insulin therapy

---

DM, diabetes mellitus; ATP, adenosine triphosphate; GI, gastrointestinal

EXPLANATION: PHARMACOLOGICAL MANAGEMENT OF DIABETES MELLITUS

Patients with type 1 DM always require administration of **insulin**. In type 2 DM, sometimes diet restriction is enough, other patients require oral hypoglycaemics, and some require insulin therapy.

Oral hypoglycaemics that may be prescribed include:

- **Sulphonylureas** (e.g. gliclazide and glibenclamide) – **increase insulin release** from beta cells by inhibiting the ATP-sensitive K^+ channel in the beta cell membrane
- **Biguanides** (e.g. metformin) – act peripherally to **increase glucose uptake** and reduce hepatic glucose output. Their mechanism of action is not understood but they do not increase insulin release
- **Alpha-glucosidase inhibitors** (e.g. acarbose) – inhibit alpha-glucosidase and therefore the digestion of starch, so blood glucose does not shoot up after a meal (**post-prandial**)
- **Thiazolidinediones** (e.g. rosiglitazone) – a new class of oral hypoglycaemics that decrease insulin resistance. They are used in conjunction with insulin therapy.

Insulin administration inhibits glucose production and reduces glucose uptake. There are three main types of insulin preparation:

- Short-acting
- Intermediate-acting
- Long-acting.

Usually a **mixed preparation** is used (for example, Mixtard 30 which is 30% short-acting and 70% intermediate-acting insulin).

The dose of insulin is **adjusted** on an individual basis by gradually increasing the dose. Insulin requirements may be **increased** by infection, stress, accidental or surgical trauma, puberty and pregnancy. **Insulin is inactivated** by GI enzymes, so must be given by **injection** – usually subcutaneous (39).

Answers

38. 1 – B, 2 – C, 3 – A, 4 – D, 5 – B
39. See explanation
40. F F T F T

41. Give three factors that should be controlled in order to reduce the complications of diabetes mellitus

42. Diabetic patients have

a. Raised high-density lipoprotein cholesterol
b. Raised triglycerides
c. An increased risk of cardiovascular disease
d. An increased risk of limb ischaemia
e. A decreased risk of cataracts

43. Describe the chronic complications of diabetes mellitus

ACE, angiotensin-converting enzyme; DM, diabetes mellitus; LDL, low-density lipoprotein; TAG, triglyceride

EXPLANATION: COMPLICATIONS OF DIABETES MELLITUS

To obtain **good control** over the **complications** of diabetes the following must be achieved (41):

- Control of blood glucose
- Control of **hyperlipidaemia** (lipid-regulating drugs can be given)
- Control of **blood pressure** (130/80 – tight blood pressure control reduces macro- and microvascular disease and mortality – use an ACE inhibitor drug).

Acute complications include **hypoglycaemia** (as a result of incorrect management) and **ketoacidosis** (characterized by dehydration, air hunger, smell of ketones, vomiting and abdominal pain).

Chronic complications of DM can be either macrovascular or microvascular (43).

MACROVASCULAR This is atherosclerotic disease affecting medium and large blood vessels. It covers:

- Cardiovascular disease – There is a two- to four-fold increase in cardiovascular disease in diabetic patients, independent of other risk factors. Diabetic patients have raised LDL-cholesterol and raised TAGs
- Renovascular disease (**impaired renal function**) – this involves increased excretion of albumin and is associated with cardiovascular disease (hypertension, myocardial infarction, coronary heart disease), the incidence of which is about 15-fold greater in patients with diabetic nephropathy
- Cerebrovascular disease – stroke
- Peripheral vascular disease – resulting in limb ischaemia due to reduced blood supply
- Neuropathy – loss of sensation increases risk of accidental trauma.

MICROVASCULAR

- Retinopathy – this is a microvascular disease that leads to capillary occlusion, interrupting the blood supply to the retina
- Cataracts.

Answers
41. See explanation
42. F T T T F
43. See explanation

DEVELOPMENT AND AGEING OF THE REPRODUCTIVE TRACTS

4 — DEVELOPMENT AND AGEING OF THE REPRODUCTIVE TRACTS

1. Concerning sexual determination and early sexual differentiation

a. Male sex is determined by the sex-determining region on the X chromosome
b. The default pathway of sexual differentiation is male
c. Androgens determine testis formation
d. Sertoli cells secrete anti-mullerian hormone
e. Testosterone is involved in the development of the male genital ductal system

2. Concerning the internal genital tracts

a. Both male and female embryos initially contain similar primordial duct systems
b. Until week 8 of gestation, male and female reproductive tracts develop along an identical course
c. The paramesonephric ducts give rise to the epididymis and vasa deferentia
d. The mesonephric ducts develop into the fallopian tubes, uterus and superior part of the vagina
e. Abnormal fusion of the mullerian ducts may result in a bifurcate uterus

3. Match the following male and female anatomical structures with the indifferent genitalia below

Options

A. Genital tubercle
B. Urogenital slit
C. Urethral fold
D. Labioscrotal swelling

1. Scrotum
2. Clitoris
3. Labium minus
4. Urethral meatus
5. Glans penis
6. Labium majus

AMH, anti-mullerian hormone; SRY, sex-determining region on the Y chromosome

EXPLANATION: SEXUAL DIFFERENTIATION

Genes on the **Y** chromosome are directly responsible for determining gender. It is the **sex-determining region on the Y chromosome (*SRY*) gene** that induces **testis formation** and it is the absence of this region in a female embryo that results in the **development of the female reproductive tract**, along a **default** pathway. This is why **XY** individuals are normally **male** and **XX** individuals are normally **female**.

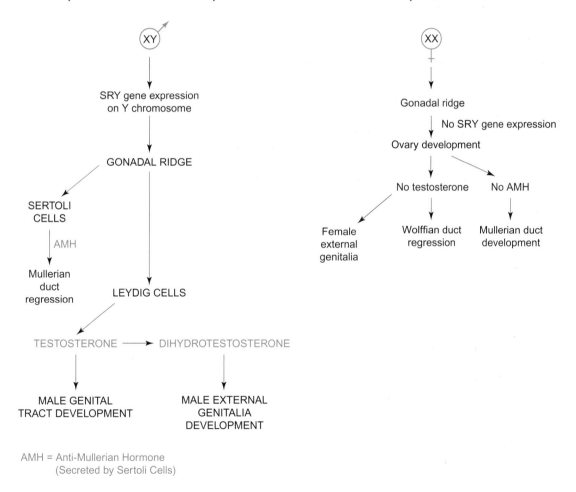

AMH = Anti-Mullerian Hormone
(Secreted by Sertoli Cells)

The time course of embryological development is explained on page 94.

Answers
1. F F F T T
2. T F F F T See text on page 94
3. 1 – D, 2 – A, 3 – C, 4 – B, 5 – A, 6 – D See diagram on page 94

4. Concerning the initiation of puberty

    a. The gonads are responsible for the initial rise in circulating androgens

    b. Growth hormone and thyroid-stimulating hormone contribute to the adolescent growth spurt

    c. Maturation of hypothalamic control mechanisms occurs

    d. Adrenal androgens provoke pubic and axillary hair growth in the early stages of puberty

    e. Growth hormone stimulates sex steroid secretion by the gonads

5. With regard to pubertal changes in the female

    a. Thelarche occurs approximately 2 years after menarche

    b. Adrenarche is the earliest developmental event

    c. Menarche signals the start of ovulatory menstrual cycles

    d. Breast growth and development does not occur until menarche

    e. Includes the keratinization of the vaginal mucosa

6. Pubertal changes in the male

    a. Adrenarche stimulates the development of pubic hair

    b. Testicular maturation occurs prior to adrenarche

    c. Seminiferous tubules grow and develop

    d. Spermatogenesis begins

    e. Testicular androgens are secreted from the Leydig cells

---

GH, growth hormone; TSH, thyroid-stimulating hormone; ACTH, adrenocorticotrophic hormone; GnRH, gonadotrophin-releasing hormone

EXPLANATION: PUBERTY

In both males and females, hypothalamic maturation during late childhood results in raised levels of GH, TSH and ACTH. **ACTH stimulates the adrenal cortex to produce sufficient amounts of adrenal androgens required for initiating pubic and axillary hair growth – adrenarche**. Girls with ACTH deficiency may go through the gonadotrophic events of puberty normally but develop no pubic hair. Boys have sufficient testicular testosterone to make up for the loss of adrenal androgen secretion. **Increased GnRH**, initially secreted more at night, **stimulates LH and FSH secretion which in turn stimulates gonadal growth**. The subsequent **rise in gonadal sex steroids prompts the development of secondary sexual characteristics**. GH, TSH and sex steroids are responsible for the adolescent growth spurt.

The **initiation of puberty** is not fully understood but it is at least partly dependent on energy status, with body weight, fat mass, nutritional status and exercise all playing a role.

Female	Male
Adrenarche: Growth spurt begins, lasts approx. 2–3 years. Pubic and axillary hair growth	**Adrenarche**: Growth spurt begins, lasts approx. 2–3 years. Pubic and axillary hair growth
Thelarche: Breast development, nipple enlargement, pigmentation and fat deposition	**Testicular maturation**: Involves initiation of androgen production by Leydig cells, seminiferous tubule growth and initiation of spermatogenesis
Menarche: Menstruation begins. Approx. 90 per cent of menstrual cycles are anovulatory in the first year of menarche and the frequency of ovulatory cycles gradually increases with age	
Secondary sexual characteristics: • Pubic and axillary hair • Breast growth and development • Enlargement of labia minora, majora + uterus • Keratinization of vaginal mucosa • Increased fat deposition in thighs, hips	**Secondary sexual characteristics**: • Pubic and axillary hair • Testicular and penile enlargement • Increased hair on trunk, pubis, axillae, face • Increased laryngeal size, deepening of voice • Increased bone and muscle mass

Answers
4. F T T T F
5. F T F F T
6. T F T T T

7. With regard to the condition of secondary hermaphroditism

   a. It results from a failure of a hormone response in the genitalia
   b. Testicular feminization syndrome is due to an increased sensitivity of fetal genitalia to oestrogen
   c. The genotype is XXY
   d. Female external genitalia and intra-abdominal testes are present in testicular feminization syndrome
   e. Insensitivity to androgens results in little pubic or axillary hair growth

8. Outline the main causes of delayed puberty in the male and female

AMH, anti-Mullerian hormone; GnRH, gonadotrophin-releasing hormone; LH, luteinizing hormone; FSH, follicle-stimulating hormone; CNS, central nervous system

EXPLANATION: ABNORMALITIES OF SEXUAL DIFFERENTIATION AND PUBERTY

Failure in endocrine communication between the gonads (ovaries and testes), and internal and external genitalia can result in a mismatch between gonadal and genital sex causing the condition of secondary (or pseudo) hermaphroditism. An example of this is **testicular feminization syndrome** (also called androgen-insensitivity syndrome). **The genotype is XY (male).** Testes develop normally due to the presence of the *SRY* gene and produce testosterone and AMH. However, these individuals are **genetically insensitive to androgens** because they have a lack of functional androgen receptors and there is a regression of the Wolffian ducts. The mullerian ducts have already regressed due to the presence of AMH. The external genitalia cannot respond to circulating androgens. Thus, this genetically male individual has intra-abdominal testes but appears female with labia, clitoris and vagina. There is little or no pubic and axillary hair and the individual is infertile.

Delayed puberty may be defined as the absence of secondary sexual characteristics by the age of 13 years in the female and 16 years in the male. There are three main causes of pubertal delay (8):

- **Constitutional delay** (includes growth delay) may only be diagnosed in an individual in the absence of pathology and thus may be **considered 'normal'** for that individual. A positive family history of delayed puberty is usually present
- **Hypogonadotrophic hypogonadism** occurs due to **deficiencies in pulsatile GnRH, LH or FSH**. GnRH deficiencies may occur as a result of genetic and developmental defects of the hypothalamus or destructive lesions of the hypothalamus or pituitary stalk. Intense exercise may also delay puberty due to inhibition of GnRH secretion. CNS tumours are the main cause of LH and FSH deficiencies
- **Hypergonadotrophic hypogonadism** occurs most commonly due to **primary gonadal failure**, resulting in decreased or failed gonadal steroid secretion. The lack of testicular or ovarian steroids causes increased FSH and LH secretion due to the lack of negative feedback. Examples of primary gonadal failure include **Klinefelter's syndrome, Turner's syndrome, mosaicism** and congenital adrenal hyperplasia.

Answers

7. T F F T T
8. See explanation

9. Outline the structure of an ovary

10. Concerning gametogenesis

a. All potential gametes in the female are produced before birth
b. The loss of many oocytes occurs during childhood
c. Women enter puberty with approximately two million oogonia remaining
d. Primary oocytes continue to develop throughout childhood
e. Post puberty, there is regular recruitment of follicles into the pool of growing follicles

11. A Graafian follicle

a. Is the final stage of the development of the primary follicle
b. Is under the influence of luteinizing hormone
c. Ruptures on day 12 of the menstrual cycle
d. Normally contains only one oocyte at any one time
e. Develops into the corpus luteum only once the ovum has been fertilized

12. Arrange the following stages of oogenesis to match with the correct statement

Options

A. Produces the division of the oocyte and the first polar body
B. Produces a haploid gamete and the second polar body
C. Increases the number of potential eggs
D. Occurs during follicular growth

1. The LH surge
2. Fertilization
3. Miltoses of oogonia
4. Growth of the oocyte

LH, luteinizing hormone

EXPLANATION: OOGENESIS

Gametogenesis differs dramatically between males and females. In the female, mitosis of oogonia terminates well before birth. Women are therefore born with all the oocytes they will ever have (approx. two million). **Primary oocytes** arrest in their development and many degenerate until puberty is reached (approx. only 400 000 oocytes may remain by the time puberty is reached). Oocytes are contained in primordial follicles. Regular recruitment of these follicles into a pool of growing follicles occurs after puberty. The sequence of steps involved in the development of an ovum (oogenesis) is shown below.

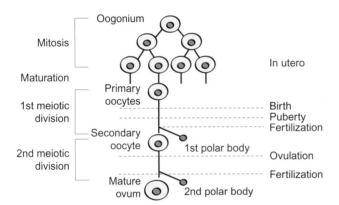

Definitions:

- **Haploid**: each set of chromosomes is called a haploid set
- **Diploid**: 23 pairs of homologous chromosomes, i.e. 46 chromosomes.

The diagram below shows the **structure of an ovary** (9).

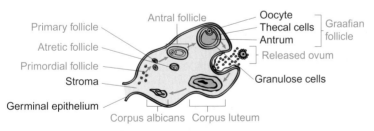

The **Graafian follicle** contains one oocyte per follicle. On about **day 14** of the menstrual cycle, in response to the **LH surge**, the epithelium and granulosa cell surface of the ovary rupture. The oocyte is released into the peritoneal cavity and **is** collected by the cilia on the fimbria of the fallopian tubes. The ruptured follicle forms the **corpus luteum**, which in the non-pregnant female regresses after approximately **10 days**. In the pregnant female, the corpus luteum continues to secrete progesterone until the placenta takes over this role.

Answers
9. See explanation
10. T T F F T
11. T T F T F
12. 1 – A, 2 – B, 3 – C, 4 – D

13. Draw a diagram to illustrate the communication between the hypothalamus and the ovary

14. Regarding gonadotrophin-releasing hormone

   a. The hypothalamus releases gonadotrophin-releasing hormone in pulses
   b. Higher neural centres regulate the hypothalamus
   c. Gonadotropes are found in the posterior pituitary
   d. Gonadotrophin-releasing hormone stimulates luteinizing hormone and follicle-stimulating hormone secretion
   e. Gonadotrophin-releasing hormone secretion increases at puberty

15. Regarding feedback mechanisms

   a. Gonadotropin secretion increases when oestrogen levels are low
   b. Plasma luteinizing hormone and follicle-stimulating hormone levels decrease after the menopause
   c. Oestrogen may exert a positive feedback effect on luteinizing hormone secretion
   d. Progesterone exerts negative feedback on the anterior pituitary during the luteal phase
   e. High plasma oestrogen levels may cause ovulation at any point in the menstrual cycle

GnRH, gonadotrophin-releasing hormone; LH, luteinizing hormone; FSH, follicle-stimulating hormone

EXPLANATION: HYPOTHALAMIC CONTROL OF GONADAL FUNCTION IN THE FEMALE

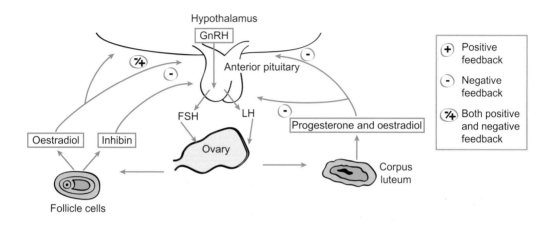

The cells of the **hypothalamus** receive signals from higher centres in the brain, generate neural signals of their own and have a neuroendocrine function. GnRH is released as a series of pulses into the portal vessels; binds to receptors on the gonadotropes in the **anterior pituitary** and drives LH secretion (and to a lesser extent FSH) in a similar pulsatile fashion. Therefore a change in GnRH pulse frequency affects the secretion of LH and FSH.

Negative and positive feedback mechanisms are important to understand.

1. **Oestradiol** exerts both a **positive** and a **negative feedback** effect on the anterior pituitary.
   - If oestradiol levels are low, **negative feedback is low, and FSH and LH secretion rises**, thus stimulating the production of oestrogen from the ovary. As oestrogen levels rise, the effect of negative feedback upon the anterior pituitary reduces FSH and LH secretion. The increase in plasma FSH and LH following ovariectomy or the menopause demonstrates this best, and an infusion of oestrogen results in the rapid decline of FSH and LH levels.
   - However, under some circumstances, **oestradiol can exert a 'positive' feedback effect**. For example, if oestrogen concentrations remain high for 48 hours or so (as seen at the end of the follicular phase of the menstrual cycle), FSH and LH secretion is enhanced, not suppressed. Thus, the LH surge occurs.
2. **Progesterone** exerts a **negative feedback** effect on the anterior pituitary. During the luteal phase of the menstrual cycle, progesterone enhances the negative feedback effects of oestrogen, LH and FSH levels are kept low and the growth of new follicles is limited. As steroid hormone levels fall at the end of the luteal phase, negative feedback is reduced and LH and FSH levels rise, stimulating a new wave of follicular growth.

Answers
13. See diagram
14. T T F T T
15. T F T T F

16. **In relation to a normal fertile menstrual cycle, which of the following statements are correct**

Options

    a. Basal body temperature rises shortly before ovulation
    b. The LH surge triggers ovulation
    c. Both the follicle and the corpus luteum secrete oestradiol
    d. Progesterone levels fall after the onset of menstruation
    e. Cervical mucus secretion peaks around mid-cycle

17. **Regarding the endometrium during the menstrual cycle**

    a. The endometrium has two distinct layers
    b. The stratum basale contains spiral arteries that are influenced by changing hormone levels
    c. Menstruation occurs with the constriction and necrosis of the spiral arteries
    d. Rising progesterone levels are responsible for the glandular proliferation of the endometrium
    e. The stratum basale is shed during menstruation

18. **Other changes during the menstrual cycle**

    a. The Graafian follicle develops during the luteal phase
    b. Cervical mucus increases during the follicular phase of the cycle
    c. Spinnbarkeit of mucus is present during the follicular phase
    d. Basal body temperature is affected by the phase of the menstrual cycle
    e. Body temperature rises during menstruation

19. **Menstruation**

    a. Occurs at the end of the follicular phase
    b. Occurs if fertilization does not take place
    c. Occurs in response to falling gonadotrophin levels
    d. Prompts new follicular development within the ovary
    e. Usually occurs about every 28 days

FSH, follicle-stimulating hormone; LH, luteinizing hormone

EXPLANATION: OVARIAN FUNCTION

Hormonal and other changes during the menstrual cycle are shown below.

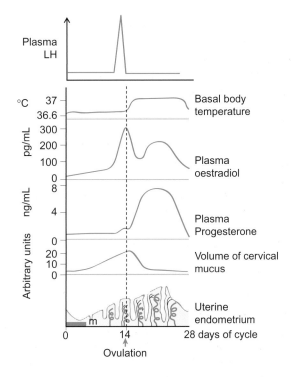

MENSTRUATION

The endometrium has two distinct layers: the **stratum basale** and **functionale**. It is the stratum functionale that is shed at menstruation, due to the constriction and necrosis of the supplying spiral arteries. The changing hormone levels bring about these changes in the arteries.

If fertilization does not occur during the luteal phase of the menstrual cycle, the **corpus luteum** cannot sustain progesterone production and disintegrates into the **corpus albicans**. The **fall in progesterone** increases the availability of prostaglandins (potent stimulators of myometrial contractility) and **menstruation begins**. The fall in steroid levels reduces the negative feedback on LH and FSH secretion, and the levels of these hormones rise, stimulating a new wave of follicular growth.

20. Outline the structure of a testis

21. Seminiferous tubules

a. Are the site of spermatogenesis
b. Contain androgen-secreting cells
c. Contain Sertoli cells that produce a blood/testis barrier
d. Store spermatids until they become motile
e. Are surrounded by blood vessels and Leydig cells

22. Concerning the sequence of spermatogenesis

a. It commences at birth
b. It produces haploid spermatozoa by meiosis from diploid spermatogonia
c. Spermatogonia undergo meiosis prior to mitosis
d. The process takes approximately 64 days in the post-pubertal male
e. Spermatids undergo extensive cell modelling as part of spermiogenesis

23. The mature spermatozoon

a. Does not become motile until it has passed through the epididymis
b. Releases sex steroids
c. Is capable of fertilization immediately after ejaculation has occurred
d. Are stored, ready for ejaculation, in the seminal vesicles
e. Contain an acrosomal cap, a mitochondrial midpiece and a tail

EXPLANATION: SPERMATOGENESIS

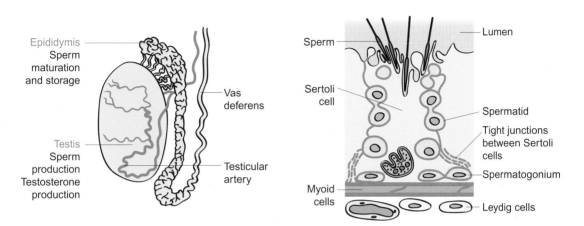

The testes have two distinct functions: **spermatogenesis** and **androgen production**. Spermatogenesis occurs within the **seminiferous tubules** and androgen production occurs in **Leydig cells** that lie in the **interstitium**. The seminiferous tubules contain the cells responsible for spermatogenesis, **Sertoli cells** and **spermatogonia**. The **Sertoli cells** perform a variety of functions. They act as a 'nurse' cell, providing metabolic and structural support for the developing spermatozoa and they form a blood/testis barrier that protects spermatogenic cells from an adverse immune response. In addition, this barrier excludes many substances present in the circulation from the seminiferous tubule fluid.

Spermatogenesis begins at puberty, in contrast to oogenesis in the female, which happens before birth. It involves three phases and takes approximately 64 days:

1. **Mitotic proliferation** to produce a large germ cell population. **Diploid** spermatogonia lie on the basement membrane of the seminiferous tubules and undergo mitotic division in order to maintain the germ cell population. **Primary spermatocytes** are the product of the final mitotic division
2. **Meiotic division** to produce genetic diversity. Primary spermatocytes undergo two meiotic divisions to halve their number of chromosomes. **Haploid spermatids** are the result of the second division. The spermatids undergo extensive cytoplasmic remodeling during the process of spermiogenesis. They develop an **acrosome**, and a **tail with a midpiece containing mitochondria**
3. **Maturation**. Spermatozoa are not fully mature as they leave the testis. Further cell membrane and cytoplasmic changes occur as they pass through the epididymis. However, it is not until they reach the female tract that they are fully capable of fertilizing an egg.

Answers

20. See diagram
21. T F T F T
22. F T F T T
23. T F F F T

24. Concerning testicular steroids

a. Androgen production occurs in Sertoli cells
b. Once synthesized, they diffuse into the circulation
c. Sertoli cells produce inhibin
d. Sex-hormone binding globulin and albumin bind testosterone in the plasma
e. Follicle-stimulating hormone secretion stimulates testosterone production in the testis

25. Draw a diagram to illustrate the hormonal control of testicular function

26. Concerning feedback control

a. Inhibin acts to suppress luteinizing hormone secretion
b. Follicle-stimulating hormone acts on the Leydig cells
c. Enhanced testosterone secretion may feedback on the anterior pituitary to decrease luteinizing hormone secretion
d. Many of the peripheral actions of testosterone are due to its conversion to dihydrotestosterone
e. Dihydrotestosterone can be metabolized to oestradiol

GnRH, gonadotrophin-releasing hormone; FSH, follicle-stimulating hormone; LH, luteinizing hormone; SHBG, sex-hormone-binding globulin

EXPLANATION: HYPOTHALAMIC CONTROL OF GONADAL FUNCTION IN THE MALE

The hormonal control of testicular function is described in the following diagram.

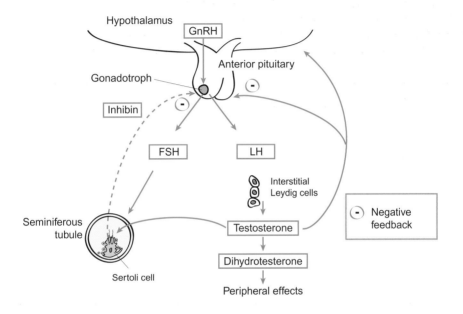

In the testes, **androgen** production occurs in the **Leydig cells**, under the influence of LH. Androgens either enter the circulation or diffuse into the Sertoli cells. Androgens feedback onto the hypothalamic–pituitary axis to inhibit LH secretion. Sertoli cells produce the hormone **inhibin**, which acts on the anterior pituitary to suppress FSH secretion.

In the circulation, 60 per cent of testosterone is transported via **SHBG** and 38 per cent by albumin. The remaining 2 per cent is free to diffuse into cells and exert an effect. Many of the peripheral responses to testosterone are due to its conversion to 5-alpha-dihydrotestosterone. Testosterone can also be metabolized to oestradiol in peripheral tissues.

Answers
24. F T T T F
25. See diagram
26. F F T T F

27. Concerning the physiological effects of progesterone

a. It is involved in breast tissue proliferation
b. It causes a decrease in the viscosity of cervical mucus during the menstrual cycle
c. It is solely responsible for pubic and axillary hair growth
d. It influences the central nervous system regulation of thermogenesis
e. It is directly responsible for ovulation

28. During pregnancy

a. Ovulation ceases
b. Oestrogen stimulates myometrial hypertrophy
c. Progesterone causes an increase in the contractility of the myometrium towards term
d. Fluid retention and an increase in uterine blood flow are due to oestrogens
e. Progesterone inhibits prepartum lactation

29. During puberty

a. Fat deposition is under the control of progesterone
b. The initiation of cyclical changes to the endometrium are influenced by oestrogen
c. Oestrogen is responsible for the closure of bone epiphyses in the female
d. Rising androgen levels stimulate facial hair growth
e. Progesterone causes a rise in basal body temperature in the luteal phase

30. Outline the physiological effects of testicular androgens in the adult male

EXPLANATION: PHYSIOLOGICAL EFFECTS OF OESTROGENS AND ANDROGENS

The tables below list the effects of progesterone and oestrogen in the female, and testosterone in the male (30).

	Effects of oestrogen	Effects of progesterone
Puberty	Stimulation of uterine, vaginal and breast tissue Proliferation of breast tissue Fat deposition Closure of epiphyses	Proliferation of breast tissue Cyclical changes to endometrium Regulates thermogenesis
Menstrual cycle	Endometrial proliferation Clear mucus secretion Maturation of vaginal epithelium	Increases body temperature Increases secretions of endometrium Thick cervical mucus production, increases pH
Pregnancy	Growth of breast duct system Myometrial hypertrophy Fluid retention Increases in uterine blood flow	Maintains decidual lining of uterus Decreases myometrial contractions and relaxes uterine smooth muscle Limits prepartum lactation Increases growth of breast alveoli

NB: Testosterone is responsible for pubic and axillary hair growth in females.

	Effects of testosterone
In the fetus	Sexual differentiation
Puberty	Pubic and axillary hair growth Penile, scrotal and muscle growth Deepening of voice Spermatogenesis Closure of long bone epiphyses (after conversion to oestradiol)
Adulthood	Hair loss Anabolic effects Maintenance of external genitalia, spermatogenesis and libido

Answers

27. T F F T F
28. T T F T T
29. F T T T T
30. See explanation

31. Sexual behaviour in humans

    a. Is solely genetically determined
    b. Is influenced by the sex steroids
    c. Begins to differentiate between girls and boys at puberty
    d. May be influenced by social stereotyping
    e. If male genitalia are present, male sexual behaviour is predetermined

32. Concerning the female and male sexual responses

    a. The male has to wait for a period of time before penile erection can occur again
    b. The female orgasm may last for a longer period of time than in the male
    c. The female has a refractory period post-ejaculation
    d. Penile erection results from the vasodilatation of penile smooth muscle
    e. Vaginal lubrication aids coitus

33. With regard to sexual dysfunction

    a. Alcohol is the commonest cause of impotence in the male
    b. It can result from a loss of libido
    c. It may be caused by diabetes mellitus
    d. Hormone replacement therapy may improve sexual dysfunction if caused by postmenopausal vaginismus
    e. It may be a result of pelvic infections in females

DM, diabetes mellitus; MS, multiple sclerosis

EXPLANATION: SEXUAL BEHAVIOUR AND RESPONSE

Human sexual behaviour is not completely understood. It is influenced by many different factors including gender, gonads, endogenous sex steroids and social stereotyping, none of which exclusively determines sexual behaviour. The rise in endogenous **hormones** at puberty acts on both the brain and the genitalia, influencing subsequent sexual behaviour. Male and female sexual responses are compared in the table below.

Phase	Male	Female
Excitement	Vasodilatation of penile smooth muscle = erection	Clitoral engorgement Vaginal lubrication
Plateau	Further vasocongestion Sperm emission into urethra	Further vasocongestion NB: May take longer to reach than in male
Orgasm	Urethral contraction = ejaculation	Rhythmic contractions of uterus NB: May last longer than male orgasm
Resolution	**First phase:** absolute refractory period. This refers to the initial period of time after ejaculation when the penis does not respond to further stimulation **Second phase:** relative refractory period. This refers to the secondary stage post-ejaculation when the penis may become excitable again with sufficient stimulation	No absolute refractory period

Causes of **sexual dysfunction** are listed in the table below.

Sexual dysfunction causes	Possible causes	Sexual dysfunction	Possible
Male		**Female**	
Loss of libido	Systemic illness Stress Fatigue Depression	Loss of libido Sexual arousal disorders	Systemic illness Medication Alcohol
Erectile dysfunction	Alcohol Drugs Endocrine disorders, e.g. DM Vascular disease, e.g. atherosclerosis Neuropathy, e.g. MS	Dyspareunia Vaginismus Anorgasmia	Infection Psychosomatic Infection

Answers
31. F T T T F
32. T T F T T
33. T T T T T

34. Ageing and fertility

a. Ageing is synonymous with the term senescence
b. Fertility is highest in women in their thirties
c. The ability to conceive decreases after the age of 35 years
d. A post-menopausal female is infertile
e. Testosterone levels decrease as men increase in age

35. Concerning the menopause

a. It is defined as the last menstrual cycle
b. Oestrogen levels decrease
c. It is often preceded by irregular cycles
d. Circulating levels of gonadotrophins decrease
e. Hot flushes and night sweats are common

36. How may menopausal symptoms be managed? Outline the benefits and risks

37. Post-menopausal bleeding

a. Is considered to be of malignant origin until proven otherwise
b. Is classified as bleeding occurring more than one year after the last menstrual cycle
c. Should always be investigated
d. Is a late sign of malignant disease
e. May be benign

HRT, hormone replacement therapy

EXPLANATION: FERTILITY CHANGES WITH AGE AND THE MENOPAUSE

Ageing begins at conception and is a description of what happens with the passage of time. **Senescence** describes deterioration related to dysfunction and disease and typically begins in middle age.

In general, women are most fertile in their twenties, declining thereafter. The capacity to conceive declines rapidly after the age of 35 years. The **menopause** marks the end of female reproductive capacity, resulting from the **exhaustion of functional ovarian follicles** and the last menstrual cycle. Oestrogen levels fall (remaining low levels of oestrogen are produced via peripheral conversion of adrenal steroids) and gonadotrophin secretion increases. Common immediate side effects of the menopause are hot flushes, night sweats, insomnia and depression. These may be relieved with the use of **HRT**.

Men do not experience a similar dramatic decrease in fertility, and spermatozoa are normally produced throughout life. However, there is a gradual decrease in testosterone production as men increase in age. Loss of libido, erectile dysfunction and failure occur with higher frequency after the age of 40 years.

The benefits and risks of HRT are summarized in the table below (36).

Benefits	Risks
Gives good and immediate symptom relief	Increases risk of thromboembolism (risk highest in first year of treatment)
Reduces risk of osteoporosis and related fractures	Increases breast cancer risk (increases with each year of use)
Reduces risk of colon cancer	Increases risk of vascular disease (e.g. heart attacks, strokes)
May reduce incidence of Alzheimer's disease	Oestrogen-only preparations increase the risk of endometrial cancer

NB: In osteoporosis there is reduced bone mass, resulting in fragile bones and an increased risk of fractures.

Post-menopausal bleeding is defined as bleeding from the genital tract occurring six months or more after the menopause. It is a serious symptom that is considered to be an early sign of malignant disease until proven otherwise. Thus it always warrants investigation. However, it may have a benign cause. Causes of post-menopausal bleeding include neoplasia of the reproductive tract, vaginitis, polyps or foreign bodies.

Answers

34. F F T T T
35. T T T F T
36. See explanation
37. T F T F T

SEXUAL DIFFERENTIATION: continued from page 73.

TIME COURSE OF EMBRYOLOGICAL DEVELOPMENT

- **Week 3**: Somatic sex cord formation (later differentiating into follicular granulosa cells in the female and Sertoli cells in the male)
- **Week 4**: Mesonephric (Wolffian) ducts develop (later developing into the vasa deferentia and epididymis in the male, whilst in the female, they regress)
- **Week 6**: Paramesonephric (mullerian) ducts develop (in the female, these later develop into the fallopian tubes, uterus and superior vagina; whilst in the male, they regress. Abnormal fusion of the mullerian ducts may result in a bifurcate uterus)
- **Week 7**: Indifferent external genitalia develop
- **Week 9**: Paramesonephric duct fusion begins
- **Week 12**: Differentiation of external genitalia begins.

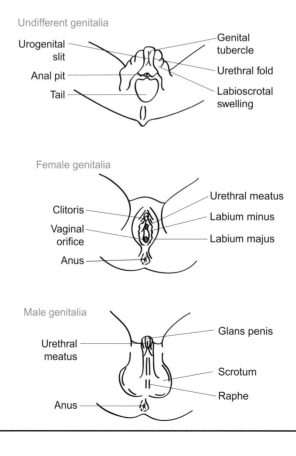

CONCEPTION, PREGNANCY AND LABOUR

SECTION 5

CONCEPTION, PREGNANCY AND LABOUR

1. Concerning capacitation of spermatozoa

a. Tail movements increase and promote sperm motility
b. It releases enzymes to dissolve the zona pellucida
c. Loss of glycoprotein molecules occurs
d. It occurs in the female genital tract
e. It follows the acrosome reaction

2. The acrosome reaction

a. Occurs after fertilization
b. Occurs within the male reproductive tract
c. Involves break down of the spermatozoan acrosome
d. Enables penetration of the zona pellucida of the oocyte
e. Is essential in order for fertilization to occur

3. Concerning fertilization

a. It involves the fusion of male and female gametes
b. The diploid state of the embryo is necessary for normal development
c. Polyspermy may be prevented by a rise in intracellular Ca^{2+} in the oocyte
d. ZP3 is initially responsible for binding the spermatozoon to the oocyte
e. It is most likely to occur in the fallopian tubes

4. Concerning subfertility in the male and female

a. Sperm defects contribute to more than 20 per cent of subfertility causes in the population
b. Failure to conceive within three months of unprotected intercourse is clinically defined as subfertility
c. Subfertility may be caused by endometriosis
d. *In vitro* fertilization always results in a viable pregnancy
e. Intracytoplasmic sperm injection is indicated in women who have decreased numbers of viable oocytes

IVF, *in vitro* fertilization; ICSI, intracytoplasmic sperm injection

EXPLANATION: FERTILIZATION

Fertilization involves the fusion of **two haploid gametes** (e.g. a sperm and an ovum) to form **one diploid zygote** (a fertilized ovum). Freshly ejaculated spermatozoa must undergo two processes before they are able to fertilize an ovum.

1. CAPACITATION This typically occurs within the female reproductive tract and involves two important events: (a) **increased tail movements** to increase motility and (b) **stripping of glycoproteins** from the spermatozoon membrane, which alters surface membrane properties. An increase in Ca^{2+} sensitivity of the spermatozoon is also seen.

2. THE ACROSOME REACTION This renders the spermatozoa capable of penetrating the **zona pellucida** of the ovum. **ZP3** on the surface membrane of the ovum binds to ZP3 receptors on the spermatozoa. This induces the spermatozoon to swell, revealing inner membranes and uncovering the ZP2 receptors. **ZP2** is responsible for the binding of the sperm and oocyte to allow penetration. This reaction must occur within close proximity to an oocyte because acrosome-reacted sperm do not survive for long.

The most common site for fertilization is within the fallopian tubes. A **rise in intracellular Ca^{2+} in the oocyte:** (a) prevents polyspermy, (b) depolarizes the egg cell membrane, (c) induces the cortical reaction and (d) induces the resumption of meiosis and expulsion of the second polar body.

Subfertility may be defined clinically as a failure to conceive within **one year** of unprotected intercourse. **Both partners** may contribute to this. Causes are compared in the following chart.

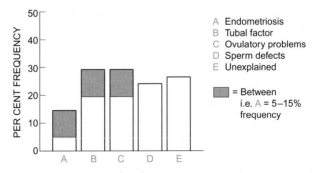

There are currently two main assisted conception techniques:

- **IVF**: This involves mixing sperm with one or more ovum, allowing fertilization and early embryo development to occur outside of the body (*in vitro*). The developing embryo is then placed in the female tract, allowing implantation to occur naturally. This procedure is referred to as one IVF cycle. Despite implementing fertilization, IVF frequently does not result in a viable pregnancy.
- **ICSI**: This involves injecting one spermatozoon into the ooplasm of the ovum *in vitro* before continuing with an IVF cycle. It is used in cases of severe **male subfertility**.

Answers
1. T F T T F
2. F F T T T
3. T T T T T
4. T F T F F

5. Concerning non-hormonal methods of contraception

    a. They may all be classified as barrier methods of contraception
    b. The natural method is most effective in women with irregular menstrual cycles
    c. The intrauterine device may remain in the uterus for up to 10 years
    d. The male condom must be placed on the flaccid penis prior to intercourse
    e. The diaphragm does not protect against infection transmission

6. Briefly outline mechanisms of producing permanent contraception in both the female and male

7. Concerning contraception in the female

    a. The combined oral contraceptive pill may prevent implantation of the fertilized ovum
    b. Depot injections result in high progestogen levels similar to those that occur in pregnancy
    c. The intrauterine device may interrupt the implantation of a fertilized ovum
    d. The progestogen-only pill blocks the luteinizing hormone surge mid-cycle, thus suppressing ovulation
    e. The combined oral contraceptive pill increases the risk of thromboembolic disease

8. Write short notes on the natural method of contraception

9. Rank the following methods of contraception in order of their failure rates, starting with the method with the highest failure rate

    A. Sterilization
    C. Male condom
    E. Implant

    B. Combined oral contraceptive pill
    D. Natural method

COCP, combined oral contraceptive pill; POP, progestogen-only pill; PMS, premenstrual syndrome; IUD, intrauterine device

EXPLANATION: CONTRACEPTION

The available non-hormonal methods of contraception are described in the following table.

	Condom	**Diaphragm**	**IUD**	**Natural** (8)	**Sterilization** (6)
Description	Latex sheath	Rubber cap used with spermicide	Small plastic or copper device	Sexual intercourse avoided during fertile period of menstrual cycle	Permanent surgical contraception
Administration	Placed over erect penis or inside vagina prior to intercourse	Fitted prior to intercourse to cover cervix	Inserted into the uterus via cervix	Measurement of basal body temperature, cervical mucus changes and ovulation timing	Bilateral vasectomy in male, fallopian tube ligation in female
Mode of action	Barrier	Barrier	Interrupts sperm migration and implantation of ovum	Prevents sperm encountering ovum	Sperm-free ejaculate, prevents oocyte encountering sperm
Failure rate per cent per hundred woman years	2–3 per cent	3–5 per cent	0.3–1 per cent	5–35 per cent	0–0.5 per cent female 0.02 per cent male
Advantages	Helps prevent infection transmission	Female is in control. Reusable	May remain in uterus up to 5 years. May be used as emergency contraception	No side effects	Permanent. Useful for those who have finished their families
Disadvantages	Requires motivation	Not protective against sexually transmitted diseases	May cause heavy periods, does not protect against infection transmission	Requires regular menstrual cycles	Permanent, risk of failure

The available hormonal methods are described in the table on page 112.

Answers
5. F F F F T
6. See explanation
7. T T T F T
8. See explanation
9. 1 – D, 2 – C, 3 – B, 4 – E, 5 – A

10. Concerning implantation

a. The embryo remains in the fallopian tube until the late morula/early blastocyst stage
b. A morula is formed from the rapidly dividing zygote
c. The syncytiotrophoblast develops into the trophoblast
d. Implantation occurs approximately 15 days post fertilization
e. Initially the trophoblast invades the endometrium

11. Concerning hormone levels in the early stages of pregnancy

a. The fertilized ovum may implant in the uterus without progesterone support
b. The corpus luteum is sustained by the release of progesterone from the developing trophoblast
c. Human chorionic gonadotrophin is produced by the trophoblast
d. The corpus luteum regresses from approximately week 7 of gestation
e. Human chorionic gonadotrophin is produced following implantation

12. Concerning the placenta

a. The syncytioblast acts as the interface between maternal and fetal blood
b. The decidua basalis lies between the myometrium and the syncytiotrophoblast
c. The umbilical cord is comprised of two umbilical veins and one umbilical artery
d. The intervillous space contains fetal blood
e. The placenta develops from the trophoblast

13. Match the following placental structures with the statements

Options

A. Carries oxygenated blood to the fetus
B. Carries deoxygenated blood to the maternal circulation
C. Lies in the decidua basalis
D. Carries maternal blood
E. Synthesizes placental hormones

1. Trophoblast
3. Umbilical artery
5. Endometrial vein
2. Umbilical vein
4. Intervillous space

hCG, human chorionic gonadotrophin

EXPLANATION: PLACENTAL STRUCTURE AND DEVELOPMENT

Embryo development and implantation are illustrated in the diagram below.

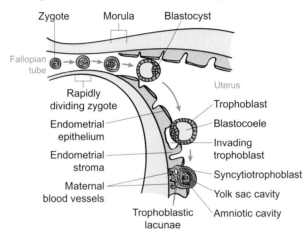

Implantation occurs approximately **6–7 days post ovulation**.

The embryo is unable to implant in the uterus without progesterone support. The **corpus luteum** produces **progesterone**, **inhibin** and **relaxin** until **week 9** of gestation, when it regresses. At this point, the developing **trophoblast** (placenta) takes over the production of progesterone. **hCG** is produced by the trophoblast following implantation and secreted into the maternal bloodstream. It acts on the corpus luteum to stimulate continued progesterone secretion.

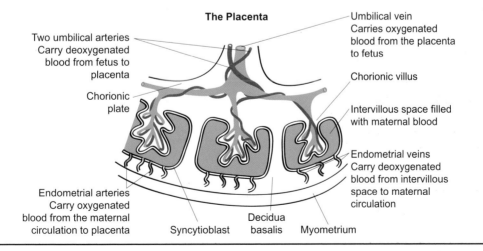

Answers

10. T T F F T
11. F F T F T
12. T T F F T
13. 1 – E, 2 – A, 3 – B, 4 – D, 5 – C

14. Concerning respiratory gas exchange in the placenta

a. Exchange of O_2 from mother to fetus occurs down a concentration gradient
b. CO_2 tension is high and O_2 tension is low in the maternal circulation
c. At the same partial pressure of O_2, saturation in fetal blood is significantly lower than that in maternal blood
d. The O_2 binding ability of fetal haemoglobin is greater than that of adult haemoglobin
e. The double Bohr effect facilitates increased O_2 transfer from mother to fetus

15. Concerning placental function

a. The placenta secretes luteinizing hormone
b. Human placental lactogen is secreted by the placenta
c. Na^+ and water are able to cross the placenta by simple diffusion
d. Amino acids may cross the placenta by special transport mechanisms
e. Maternal IgG cannot cross the placenta, whereas IgM can

16. Briefly explain the physiology of the double Bohr effect, using a diagram if required

hCG, human chorionic gonadotrophin; hPL, human placental lactogen; IgM, immunoglobulin M; IgG, immunoglobulin G

EXPLANATION: PLACENTAL FUNCTION

The placenta has **five** main functions:

1. SYNTHESIS OF HORMONES INVOLVED IN THE MAINTENANCE OF PREGNANCY The placenta secretes many **steroid** and **peptide hormones** that act locally (within the placenta) or systemically. The main placental hormones are **hCG** (until week 9 only), **progesterone**, **oestrogens** (mainly oestradiol and oestriol), **hPL** and **relaxin**.

2. RESPIRATORY GAS EXCHANGE The **partial pressure of O_2** in fetal blood is low and that of CO_2 is high when compared with maternal blood. Gradients therefore exist to drive diffusion. In addition, **fetal haemoglobin** has an increased binding ability for O_2 compared with adult haemoglobin due to a difference in haemoglobin chain morphology. The **double Bohr effect** further facilitates O_2 transfer to the fetus. A fall in the pH of maternal blood, due to uptake of fetal CO_2, drives the release of maternal O_2. The rise in fetal pH, due to the removal of CO_2, facilitates the uptake of O_2. Thus, the O_2 saturation of fetal and maternal blood is similar (see diagram) **(16)**. Note that fetal blood has a greater O_2 concentration than maternal blood at any given O_2 tension (see diagram).

3. NUTRIENT TRANSFER AND WASTE PRODUCTION **Simple diffusion** between fetal and maternal circulation facilitates the transport of low molecular weight molecules, e.g. Na^+, water, urea, fatty acids and lipid-soluble steroids. Special **transport mechanisms** exist for the transfer of complex sugars, conjugate steroids, amino acids, vitamins, plasma proteins and cholesterol.

4. HEAT TRANSFER

5. IMMUNOLOGICAL PROTECTION The placenta prevents rejection of the fetus by the maternal immune system. **Maternal IgM** cannot cross the placenta, whereas **IgG** can.

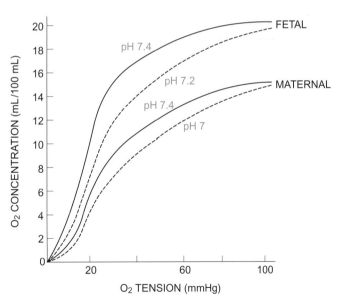

Answers

14. T F F T T
15. F T T T F
16. See explanation

17. Concerning the endocrine system during pregnancy

    a. Prolactin secretion is depressed due to increased secretion of oestrogen
    b. Circulating progesterone levels rise until term
    c. Increased placental progesterone and oestrogens prevent further follicular development
    d. Human placental lactogen release declines towards term
    e. Human chorionic gonadotrophin levels continue to rise throughout pregnancy

18. Concerning the cardiovascular system

    a. Generalized vasoconstriction occurs during pregnancy
    b. Maternal plasma volume increases
    c. Blood pressure normally decreases in pregnancy
    d. Heart rate and stroke volume increase
    e. Ejection systolic murmurs are common due to increased maternal cardiac output

19. During pregnancy

    a. The level of the diaphragm rises and the ribcage expands, causing an increase in ventilation rate
    b. Fat stores become depleted by the demands of the fetus
    c. Varicose veins and ankle oedema are common
    d. Gas exchange in the maternal lungs is increased
    e. Thromboembolism is more common than in the non-pregnant state

20. Concerning the immune system

    a. Cellular immunity increases during pregnancy
    b. Pregnant women are more susceptible to viral infections
    c. Rhesus isoimmunization may result from a rhesus-negative mother carrying a rhesus-positive child
    d. Rhesus anti-D disease may occur if a direct exchange occurs between maternal and fetal blood
    e. Maternal rhesus anti-D disease may cause a haemolytic anaemia in the fetus

---

GFR, glomerular filtration rate; T3, triiodothyronine; T4, thyroxine; TBG, thyroxine-binding globulin; HR, heart rate; SV, stroke volume; IVC, inferior vena cava; IgM, immunoglobulin M; IgG, immunoglobulin G; Rh, rhesus; hPL, human placental lactogen; hCG, human chorionic gonadotrophin

EXPLANATION: MATERNAL PHYSIOLOGY

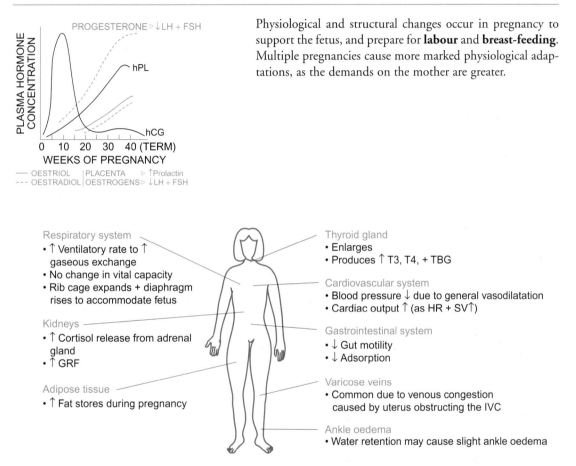

Physiological and structural changes occur in pregnancy to support the fetus, and prepare for **labour** and **breast-feeding**. Multiple pregnancies cause more marked physiological adaptations, as the demands on the mother are greater.

Respiratory system
- ↑ Ventilatory rate to ↑ gaseous exchange
- No change in vital capacity
- Rib cage expands + diaphragm rises to accommodate fetus

Kidneys
- ↑ Cortisol release from adrenal gland
- ↑ GRF

Adipose tissue
- ↑ Fat stores during pregnancy

Thyroid gland
- Enlarges
- Produces ↑ T3, T4, + TBG

Cardiovascular system
- Blood pressure ↓ due to general vasodilatation
- Cardiac output ↑ (as HR + SV↑)

Gastrointestinal system
- ↓ Gut motility
- ↓ Adsorption

Varicose veins
- Common due to venous congestion caused by uterus obstructing the IVC

Ankle oedema
- Water retention may cause slight ankle oedema

Rhesus isoimmunization occurs due to an incompatibility of maternal and fetal blood antigens. If an exchange between maternal and fetal blood occurs (e.g. during invasive procedures or at delivery) then an immune response is mounted in the form of **IgM** production. Because IgM cannot cross the placenta, the fetus is not affected. If, during a subsequent pregnancy, repeat exposure to the same red blood cell antigen occurs, then **IgG** antibodies are produced. IgG antibodies cross the placenta easily and cause red cell destruction and a **haemolytic anaemia** in the fetus. This most commonly occurs in **Rh-negative mothers** with an **Rh-positive fetus**. Rh anti-D prophylaxis may be given in these cases.

Answers
17. F T T T F
18. F T T T T
19. T F T T T
20. F T T T T

21. Concerning the first breath of life

a. It requires a large inspiratory effort by the fetus
b. Breathing movements are 'practised' *in utero* prior to parturition
c. Surfactant may be produced in fetal lungs from week 20
d. Surfactant production is stimulated by fetal corticosteroids
e. It may be prompted by light, cold and noxious stimuli

22. Match the following congenital heart defects with the correct statement

Options

A. May occur in approx. 10 per cent of adults
B. Is the most common congenital heart defect
C. May take up to a year to close in normal babies
D. Is a defect in the septum between the right and left hand side of the heart

1. Ventricular septal defect
2. Atrial septal defect
3. Patent ductus arteriosus
4. Persistent foramen ovale

23. Concerning the fetal circulation

a. The ductus arteriosus diverts blood away from the liver
b. It requires blood flow from the fetal lungs to maintain high left-sided pressures in the heart
c. The ductus venosus diverts blood away from the fetal lungs
d. The foramen ovale enables oxygenated blood to flow from the right to the left side of the heart
e. The fetal lungs are the site of gaseous exchange *in utero*

24. Briefly outline how the fetal circulation changes at birth

RA, right atrium; RV, right ventricle; LA, left atrium; LV, left ventricle; FO, foramen ovale; DA, ductus arteriosus; VSD, ventricular septal defects; PDA, patent ductus arteriosus; ASD, atrial septal defects; PS, pulmonary stenosis

EXPLANATION: FETAL AND PERINATAL PHYSIOLOGY

The fetal and adult circulations are compared in the following diagram.

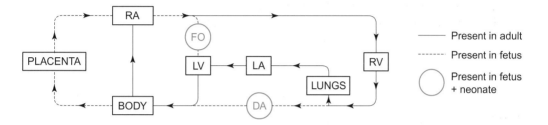

The **fetal circulation** differs from that in the adult because the organ of gaseous exchange is the **placenta and not the lungs**. The FO and DA act as **shunts**, enabling blood to bypass the developing fetal lung. This optimizes O_2 delivery. A third shunt, the ductus venosus, diverts blood away from the liver. At birth, these shunts are designed to close so that the lungs are perfused and gaseous exchange is maintained in the absence of the placenta.

During labour, the delivery of O_2 and nutrients to the fetus is reduced. This prompts the fetal circulation to pass through the lungs, causing a **drop in pressure** in the right side of the heart. The return of blood from the lungs causes **increased pressure in the left side** of the heart, **reversing the blood flow** through the DA and prompting its collapse. These pressure changes also cause the FO to close, allowing the heart to work as two pumps in series rather than one in parallel. The DA is closed permanently in most individuals by one year of age. The FO closes more slowly and remains patent in 10 per cent of adults **(24)**.

Congenital heart defects occur in approx. 8 per 1000 births. The most common include VSD (25 per cent), PDA (15 per cent), ASD (15 per cent) and PS (10 per cent).

RESPIRATORY FUNCTION CHANGES AT BIRTH

The fetus mimics breathing movements while *in utero* for reasons that are not fully understood. They may carry an element of 'practice' but also promote growth and development by distending the fetal lungs. Primitive air sacs in the lungs are present at week 20, blood vessels at week 28 and surfactant from week 30. **Surfactant** forms a surface film over the alveolus, reducing the pressure required to expand the fetal lung. Surfactant synthesis is promoted by fetal corticosteroids that rise towards delivery.

Mechanisms that may promote the **large inspiratory effort at birth** include cold and light exposure, auditory and noxious stimuli.

Answers
21. T T F T T
22. 1 – B, 2 – D, 3 – C, 4 – A
23. F F F T F
24. See explanation

25. Regarding the onset of labour

    a. It is considered to be normal if between weeks 37 and 40 of gestation
    b. Post-maturity may be defined as labour occurring after 40 weeks
    c. It is recognized by the presence of Braxton-Hicks contractions
    d. Contractions may be augmented with oxytocin
    e. Contractions increase in frequency and duration as labour progresses

26. Match one of the three stages of labour with the most appropriate statement

Options

    A. The placenta is delivered
    B. Ends at full cervical dilatation
    C. Contractions slowly subside
    D. May be initiated due to fetal hypothalamic maturation
    E. Ends with the expulsion of the fetus

    1. First stage of labour
    2. Second stage of labour
    3. Third stage of labour

27. List the hormones that are important in parturition and state their functions

EXPLANATION: LABOUR

Labour is the process by which the fetus, placenta and membranes are expelled from the uterus by co-ordinated **myometrial contractions**. This normally occurs between **37 and 42 weeks** of gestation. Premature labour occurs prior to 37 weeks and post-mature labour occurs after 42 weeks. The onset of labour may be recognized by the conversion of non-painful **Braxton-Hicks contractions** to painful, regular contractions and cervical ripening (dilatation and shortening).

The factors that trigger labour are not fully understood. A number of contributory factors may be involved:

- Increased **fetal adrenal activity**
- **Maturation** of fetal hypothalamus
- Distension of uterus stimulating **oxytocin production**
- Local production of **prostaglandins**
- Alterations in oestrogen/progesterone ratio
- Circadian rhythms.

Labour is divided into three distinct stages:

	First stage	Second stage	Third stage
Onset	Regular, painful contractions	Full cervical dilatation	Birth of the fetus
Outcome	Cervical softening and dilatation, increase in uterine contractions, fetal head descends into pelvis, membranes rupture	Fetal head engages with pelvis, uterine contractions increase, delivery of baby	Uterine contractions subside, delivery of placenta and membranes

The hormones involved in progression of labour and their functions are listed below (27).

Hormone	Function
Oestrogen	Stimulates production of oxytocin receptors in myometrium prior to labour Stimulates myometrial prostaglandin synthesis
Oxytocin	Stimulates and augments uterine contractions Stimulates prostaglandin production NB: Exogenous oxytocin can augment the first stage of labour and accelerate the third stage
Prostaglandin	Stimulates Ca^{2+} release to augment myometrial muscle contraction Involved in cervical ripening
Relaxin	Promotes pelvic ligament relaxation prior to parturition Softens cervix

Answers

25. T F F T T
26. 1 – B, D, 2 – E, 3 – C, A
27. See explanation

28. Draw a simple diagram of the female breast

29. Regarding lactation

    a. Prolactin stimulates and regulates milk production
    b. Prolactin levels rise at the onset of labour
    c. Oestrogen potentiates the action of prolactin
    d. Prolactin inhibits the production of follicle-stimulating hormone and luteinizing hormone
    e. Suckling stimulates both prolactin and oxytocin secretion

30. Using a diagram, outline the mechanism of the suckling reflex

31. Concerning breast-feeding of the infant

    a. Breast milk confers immunity to the infant
    b. Breast milk contains lipids, proteins, vitamins and immunoglobulins
    c. Colostrum is secreted for the first 4–5 days after delivery
    d. Colostrum is low in protein and high in fat
    e. Is contraindicated in mothers who are HIV positive

PRL, prolactin; IgG, immunoglobulin G; HIV, human immunodeficiency virus

EXPLANATION: THE BREAST AND LACTATION

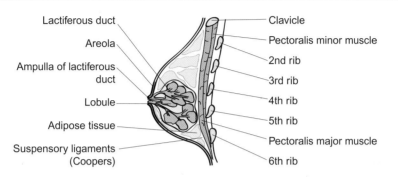

The most important hormone involved in **lactation** and the **suckling reflex** is **PRL**. Levels of PRL rise throughout pregnancy and remain high until approximately **4–6 weeks** after delivery. After this period, continued breast-feeding is necessary to stimulate the release of **prolactin** from the anterior pituitary via the suckling reflex. Suckling also induces the secretion of oxytocin from the posterior pituitary. Oxytocin acts on the mysepithelial cells of the mammary alveoli to cause milk ejection. **Progesterone and oestrogen inhibit** the action of PRL, thus lactation does not occur prior to delivery when oestrogen levels are still high.

Colostrum is secreted during late pregnancy and for the first 4–5 days after delivery. It is a thick yellow fluid that has a high protein and low fat content. **Breast milk** is composed of lipids, milk proteins, vitamins, minerals and IgG. It is high in fat, providing a source of energy.

Breast-feeding increases bonding between mother and baby, reduces the incidence of allergies in later life and leads to an improved immune system for the baby. It is not recommended for mothers who are infected with:

• HIV
• Cytomegalovirus
• Hepatitis B and/or C due to the risk of transmission from mother to baby.

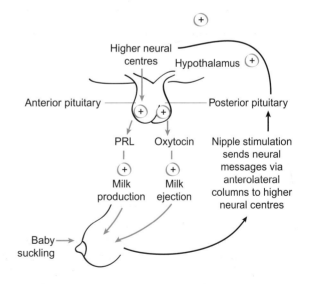

CONTRACEPTION: continued from page 99.

Hormonal methods of contraception are listed in the table below.

	COCP	POP	Depot injection	Implants
Description	Synthetic oestrogen and progestogen	Synthetic progestogen	Synthetic progestogen	Synthetic progestogen
Administration	Oral, taken for 21 days with a 7-day gap for withdrawal bleed	Oral, taken continuously at the same time every day	Intramuscular injection	Subcutaneous implantation
Mode of action	Multiple sites of action: suppression of ovulation, implantation interference	Inhibits sperm transport in cervical mucus	Suppression of ovulation	Prevents ovulation
Failure rate per cent per hundred woman years	0.2–0.3 per cent if protocol followed correctly	0.3–0.4 per cent	0–1 per cent	0–1 per cent
Advantages	May decrease PMS, menstrual bleeding, pain and acne	Useful if women cannot use COCP	Do not need to remember to take pill daily	Same as for depot
Disadvantages	Increased risk of thromboembolic disease, dyslipidaemia, hypertension	Irregular bleeding, breast discomfort, PMS, increased risk of ectopic pregnancy	Same as for POP plus weight gain and loss of bone density	Same as for POP, may be difficult to remove due to fibrosis formation

COCP, combined oral contraceptive pill; POP, progestogen-only pill; PMS, premenstrual syndrome

INDEX

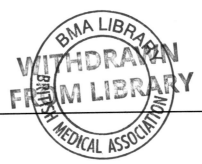